FAST FACTS

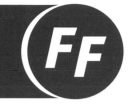

FF

Indispensable
Guides to
Clinical
Practice

D0230293

Prostate Cancer

Fourth edition

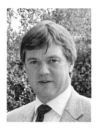

Roger S Kirby
Professor of Urology
St George's Hospital
London, UK

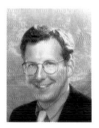

Michael K Brawer
Director, Northwest Prostate Institute
Northwest Hospital, Seattle, USA

This book is as balanced and as practical as we can make it. Ideas for
improvement are always welcome: feedback@fastfactsbooks.com

HEALTH PRESS
Oxford

Fast Facts – Prostate Cancer
First published 1996
Second edition 1998
Third edition 2001
Fourth edition March 2004

The cover design represents the division of a prostate cancer cell.

Illustrated by Dee McLean, MeDee Art, London, UK.
Typesetting and page layout by Zed, Oxford, UK.
Printed by Fine Print (Services) Ltd, Oxford, UK.

Printed with vegetable inks on fully biodegradable and
recyclable paper manufactured from sustainable forests.

444   001
Low emissions
during production

Low   Sustainable
chlorine   forests

Glossary

5α-reductase: the enzyme that converts testosterone to DHT

Antiandrogens: drugs that compete with testosterone or its metabolite DHT for binding to androgen receptors in the prostate

Brachytherapy: interstitial radiotherapy

BPH: benign prostatic hyperplasia

Cryoablation: the use of freezing temperatures to destroy tissue

CT: computerized tomography

DHT: dihydrotestosterone

DRE: digital rectal examination

EBRT: external-beam radiotherapy

EGF: epidermal growth factor

FGF: fibroblast growth factor

GM–CSF: granulocyte–macrophage colony stimulating factor

IGF: insulin-like growth factor

IPSS: International Prostate Symptom Score

LHRH antagonists: pure antagonists that shut off LHRH release obviating the flare phenomenon seen with LHRH agonists

LHRH agonists: luteinizing hormone-releasing hormone analogs, which are used to achieve androgen deprivation by inducing chemical castration. They initially stimulate the anterior pituitary resulting in a transient increase in testosterone

MRI: magnetic resonance imaging

PDGF: platelet-derived growth factor

PSA: prostate-specific antigen

TNM: tumor–nodes–metastasis (a staging system for prostate cancer)

TRUS: transrectal ultrasonography

TURP: transurethral resection of the prostate

Introduction

Although prostate cancer has long been considered the province of the hospital specialist, it is increasingly impinging on the domain of the primary care physician. Awareness of this insidious and highly prevalent disease among the general public has recently risen sharply as a result of escalating media attention, and this is encouraging more men to visit their family physician to seek the reassurance of a prostate health check. The pros and cons of prostate-specific antigen (PSA) testing now have to be explained to these individuals, including the consequences of a diagnosis of early prostate cancer, which includes the possibility of complete cure, but also the risk of side effects, such as erectile and urinary dysfunction.

Although most patients suspected of having prostate cancer will be referred to hospital for histological confirmation of the diagnosis and staging by means of a bone scan, increasingly the family physician is requested to prescribe the continuing androgen ablation therapy that so many of the sufferers from this malignancy eventually require.

The family physician is also called upon from time to time to provide counseling support, not only to the patient, but also to his sometimes distressed immediate family. Although a gratifying 80% or so of patients respond to therapy in the first instance, this response is often regrettably short-lived and disease relapse occurs, requiring second-line therapies, which are looking increasingly promising. The family physician will often be the linchpin in the organization of support services to help the patient and his family through the sometimes difficult, and often prolonged, terminal phases of the disease.

This fourth edition of *Fast Facts – Prostate Cancer* concisely delivers the evidence-based information that urologists and family physicians need today to advise, support and manage optimally their patients with prostate cancer.

In most developed and developing countries, prostate cancer is the most commonly diagnosed malignancy affecting men beyond middle age, and is second only to lung cancer as a cause of cancer deaths in men. Prostate cancer is predicted to become the principal cancer killer in men by 2006. It has been estimated that, in western countries, the lifetime risk of developing microscopic prostate cancer is approximately 30%. However, as many of these cancers grow so slowly, the risk of developing clinical disease is about 10%; the lifetime risk of actually dying from prostate cancer is approximately 3%. Worldwide, there has been a consistent increase in the incidence of clinically significant disease in recent years. Moreover, because prostate cancer is primarily a disease affecting men over the age of 50 years, the worldwide trend towards an aging population (Figure 1.1) means that the number of men at risk of death from prostate cancer is predicted to increase

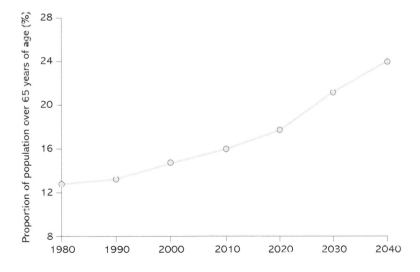

Figure 1.1 As a result of the trend towards an aging population, shown here, the incidence of prostate cancer seems likely to continue to increase worldwide.

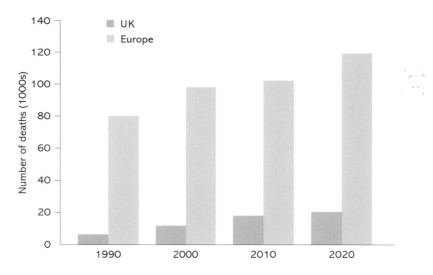

Figure 1.2 An increase in prostate cancer deaths in Europe is predicted over the next two decades as a result of population aging. Data from Boyle P. Trends in cancer mortality in Europe. *Eur J Cancer* 1992;28:7–8.

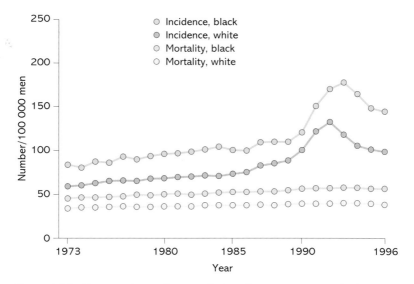

Figure 1.3 Incidence and mortality rates for invasive prostate cancer in the United States by race, 1973–1996. Note the temporary apparent rise in incidence soon after the introduction of PSA testing. Source: National Cancer Institute. *SEER Cancer Statistics Review*.

markedly during the next two decades (Figure 1.2). However, mortality in the USA has recently started to decline (Figure 1.3). Some have attributed this drop to the early detection efforts made in North America, although several other factors may also have contributed.

Risk factors

Despite the high incidence of prostate cancer, relatively little is known about the fundamental causes of the disease. However, a number of risk factors have been established (Table 1.1).

Aging. Age is the greatest factor influencing the development of prostate cancer. Clinical disease is rather rare in men below the age of 50 years, and the incidence increases markedly in men aged over 60 years of age (Figure 1.4). Microscopic foci of prostate cancer are present in 30% of men in their 50s, and in 70% of men over the age of 80 years, but many of these seem never to progress.

Race. There are marked geographical and ethnic variations in the incidence of clinical prostate cancer. The risk is highest in North America and northern European countries, and lowest in the Far East (Figure 1.5). In the USA, the risk is higher in blacks than in whites, and blacks also appear to develop the disease earlier. Chinese and Japanese races show the lowest incidence of prostate cancer. The incidence of latent disease, however, is similar in all populations studied. In migration studies, the incidence of prostate cancer in men emigrating from a low- to high-risk area increases to that of the local population within two generations.

TABLE 1.1

Recognized and possible risk factors for prostate cancer

• Aging	• 5α-reductase activity
• Race	• High-fat 'Western' diet
• Family history	• Low exposure to sunlight
• Androgens	• Environmental factors

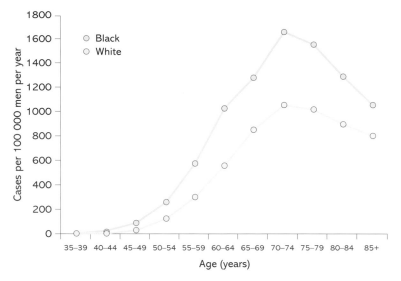

Figure 1.4 Age-specific incidence of prostate cancer in blacks and whites (US SEER program 1995–1999).

Family history. The risk of prostate cancer is increased between two- and threefold in men with a first-degree relative in whom prostate cancer was diagnosed at an early age, and increases further still when there is more than one first-degree relative with a history of prostate cancer. It is estimated that approximately 9% of all cases of prostate cancer have a genetic basis, and a hereditary prostate cancer (HPC) gene that may be responsible has now been localized to a region of the short arm of chromosome 1q. A further susceptibility gene has been identified on the X chromosome. Several other loci are currently under investigation.

Hormones. Testosterone and its more potent metabolite dihydrotestosterone (DHT) are essential for normal prostate growth, and thus may also play a role in the development of prostate cancer (Figure 1.6). Prostate cancer almost never develops in men castrated before puberty, or in individuals deficient in 5α-reductase (the enzyme, existing in type I and II isoforms, that converts testosterone to DHT). Although there is no correlation between circulating androgen concentrations and the risk of prostate cancer, the lowest quartile for serum testosterone in a population has been shown to have a decreased incidence of prostate cancer while the individuals in the highest quartile have a greater incidence. A raised 5α-reductase level may be associated with a higher incidence of the disease. At present, however, the precise role of androgens and estrogens in the development of prostate cancer remains to be established. One of the major confounders is the wide range of serum testosterone levels in 'normal' men. Other problems include lack of understanding of the active form of androgen in the prostate, quality control and specimen stability issues, and biological variability. Moreover, the true relationship between serum and prostate androgen levels may be dynamic. Finally, the age at which androgens have their greatest effect may not be the time of study measurement.

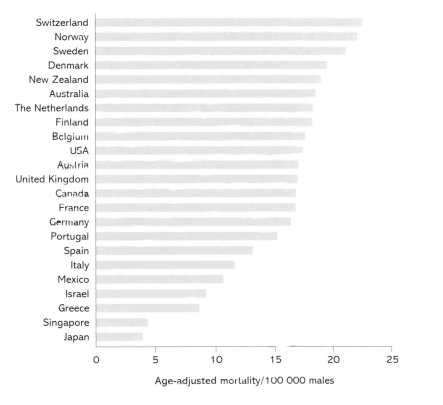

Figure 1.5 Age-adjusted mortality by country per 100 000 males.

Adapted from Parker et al. 1996.

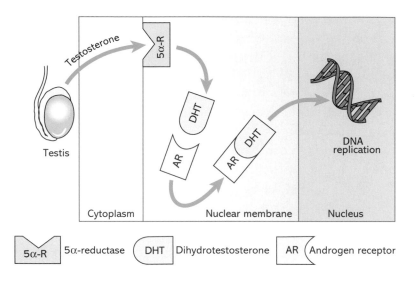

Figure 1.6 Testosterone supports prostate cell function and stimulates cell division.

Diet and chemoprevention. There is a correlation between the incidence of prostate cancer and consumption of saturated fat or red meat. This may conceivably be related to the production of free radicals or to reduced vitamin A absorption, which leads to a reduction in circulating β-carotene levels; β-carotene appears to protect against the development of certain cancers. Diets in many Asian countries, where the incidence of prostate cancer is low, contain high levels of vitamin A, in addition to phytoestrogens and other substances with biological properties that may confer anticarcinogenic activity. The incidence of prostate cancer in Japan and China is currently increasing, and it has been suggested that this is associated with the increasing adoption of a 'Western' diet. It has recently been suggested that regular intake of the antioxidant vitamin E or of selenium may protect against prostate cancer (see page 90). In a recent preliminary, randomized study, regular intake of selenium reduced prostate cancer incidence by 40%. Selenium and vitamin E are the subjects of a major chemoprevention trial now taking place in the USA. Lycopenes, which are present in tomatoes, have also been reported to have a chemopreventative effect in this disease.

Very recently, the 5α-reductase inhibitor finasteride has been shown to reduce the incidence of prostate cancer by 24.8% compared with placebo over a 7-year period, though at the cost of a small incidence of sexual side effects (see page 91). Counterbalancing this observation, those cancers that did occur in the finasteride group tended to appear more aggressive in nature. The explanation for this is still debated, but it could be an artifact resulting from the Gleason scoring system (see below), which has never been validated in patients treated by androgen deprivation.

Environmental and occupational factors. Various environmental factors related to industrial chemicals have been identified as potential promoters of prostate cancer. There is evidence to suggest that men exposed to cadmium and men working in the nuclear power industry have an increased risk of prostate cancer. There is also evidence that patients who are exposed to low levels of ultraviolet light may also be at increased risk. Indeed, in the USA, the prevalence of prostate cancer is greater in the north than in the south, and in other countries prostate cancer incidence increases in direct relation to the distance from the equator. This could conceivably be due to a protective effect of vitamin D related to exposure to sunlight.

Histological features

Most prostate cancers (> 70%) are adenocarcinomas that appear to arise in the peripheral zone of the gland (Figure 1.7). Approximately 5–15% arise in the central zone, and the remainder from the transition zone, which is where benign prostatic hyperplasia (BPH) also develops.

Microscopic foci of 'latent' prostate cancer are a common autopsy finding and may appear very early in life; approximately 30% of men over 50 years of age have evidence of latent disease. Due to the very slow growth rate of these microscopic tumors, many may never progress to clinical disease. Beyond a certain size, however, these lesions progressively dedifferentiate, owing to clonal selection, and become increasingly invasive. A tumor that has a volume greater than 0.5 cm^3 or is anything other than well differentiated is generally regarded as clinically significant.

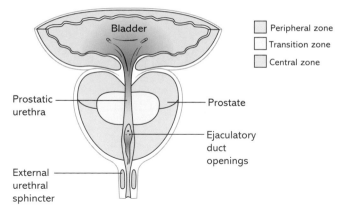

Peripheral zone
Transition zone
Central zone

Bladder

Prostatic urethra

Prostate

Ejaculatory duct openings

External urethral sphincter

Frontal view of normal prostate

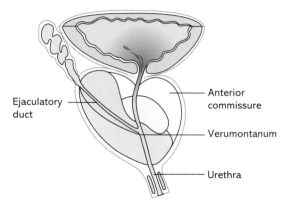

Ejaculatory duct

Anterior commissure

Verumontanum

Urethra

Sagittal view of normal prostate

Figure 1.7 Approximately 70% of prostate cancers arise in the peripheral zone.

The Gleason system is the most widely used for grading prostate cancer (Figure 1.8). It recognizes five levels of increasing aggressiveness.

- Grade 1 tumors consist of small, uniform glands with minimal nuclear changes.
- Grade 2 tumors have medium-sized acini, still separated by stromal tissue, but more closely arranged.
- Grade 3 tumors, the most common finding, show marked variation in glandular size and organization, and generally infiltration of stromal and neighboring tissues.

- Grade 4 tumors show marked cytological atypia with extensive infiltration.

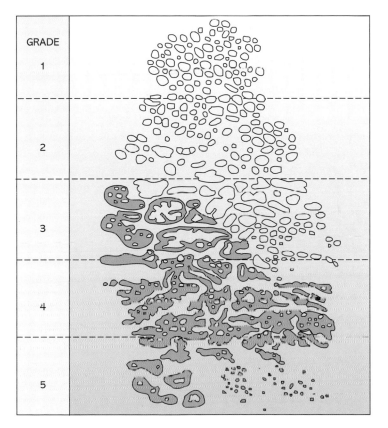

Figure 1.8 The Gleason grading system is based on the extent to which the tumor cells are arranged into recognizably glandular structures. Grade 1 tumors form almost normal glands that are progressively lost through the grades. By grade 5, tumors are characterized by sheets of undifferentiated cancer cells. In individual patients, the prognosis worsens with the progressive loss of glandular differentiation. Because prostate cancers are often heterogeneous in histological pattern, the Gleason score (or sum) is calculated by the summation of the grades of the two predominant areas. Gleason DF. The Veterans' Administration Cooperative Urologic Research Group: Histologic grading and clinical staging of prostatic carcinoma. In Tannenbaum M, ed. *Urologic Pathology: The Prostate.* Philadelphia: Lea and Febiger, 1977:171–98.

- Grade 5 tumors are characterized by sheets of undifferentiated cancer cells.

Because prostatic cancers are often heterogeneous, the numbers of the two most widely represented grades are added together to produce the Gleason score (e.g. 3 + 4) (Table 1.2). This score (or sum) provides useful prognostic information; Gleason scores above 4 are associated with a progressive risk of more rapid disease progression, increased metastatic potential and decreased survival. A meta-analysis of patients being managed by active surveillance (watchful waiting), for example, found that the annual rate of developing metastases was 2.1% in patients with Gleason scores of less than 4, compared with 5.4% in patients with scores between 5 and 7, and 13.5% in patients with scores above 7. The chance of relapse after radical prostatectomy has also been shown to be directly proportional to the percentage of Gleason grade 4 and 5 cancer in the specimen.

One study of 767 men with localized prostate cancer reported a highly significant correlation between the Gleason score and the risk of dying from prostate cancer. Patients with a score of 2–4 had a 4–7% chance of dying within 15 years of diagnosis. In contrast, patients with a score of 8–10 had a 60–87% chance of death from prostate cancer.

Patterns of disease spread

Prostate cancer can be classified according to the spread of the disease by the tumor–nodes–metastasis (TNM) system (Table 1.3). The tumor stage (T1–T4) describes the pathological development of the tumor. T1

TABLE 1.2

The Gleason score*

Gleason score	Histological characteristics	Ten-year likelihood of local progression (%)
≤ 4	Well differentiated	25
5–7	Moderately differentiated	50
> 7	Poorly differentiated	75

*The Gleason score is the sum of the two most prominent grades

TABLE 1.3

The TNM classification of prostate cancer (1997)

Primary tumor

Tx   Primary tumor cannot be assessed

T0   No evidence of primary tumor

T1   Clinically inapparent tumor not palpable or visible by imaging

      T1a   Tumor incidental; histological finding in 5% or less of tissue resected

      T1b   Tumor incidental; histological finding in more than 5% of tissue resected

      T1c   Tumor identified by needle biopsy (e.g. because of elevated PSA)

T2   Tumor confined within the prostate*

      T2a   Tumor involves one lobe

      T2b   Tumor involves both lobes

T3   Tumor extends through the prostatic capsule†

      T3a   Extracapsular extension (unilateral or bilateral)

      T3b   Tumor invades seminal vesicle(s)

T4   Tumor is fixed or invades adjacent structures other than seminal vesicles: bladder neck, external sphincter, rectum, levator muscles and/or pelvic wall

Regional lymph nodes

Nx   Regional lymph nodes cannot be assessed

N0   No regional lymph node metastasis

N1   Regional lymph node metastasis

Distant metastasis**

Mx   Distant metastasis cannot be assessed

M0   No distant metastasis

M1   Distant metastasis

      M1a   Non-regional lymph node(s)

      M1b   Bone(s)

      M1c   Other site(s)

*Tumor found in one or both lobes by needle biopsy, but not palpable or visible by imaging, is classified as T1c
†Invasion into the prostatic apex or into (but not beyond) the prostatic capsule is not classified as T3, but as T2
**When more than one site of metastasis is present, the most advanced category should be used

represents 'incidental' status, in which the tumor is discovered after transurethral resection of the prostate (TURP) or more commonly by PSA testing, and is not detectable by palpation or ultrasonography. T2 and T3 are intermediate stages; T4 represents advanced disease, in which the tumor invades neighboring organs (Figure 1.9). The nodal stages (N0–N1) and metastatic stages (M0–M1c) reflect the clinical progression of the disease. Metastases are most common in the lymph nodes (N1) and bones (M1); less commonly, the lungs and other soft tissues may also be involved.

Currently, it is not possible to distinguish unambiguously between those tumors that will remain latent throughout the patient's life and

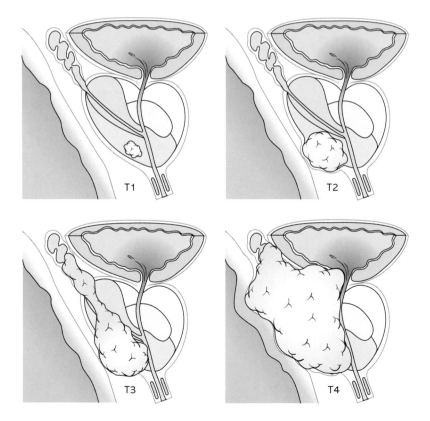

Figure 1.9 The TNM system recognizes four stages of local tumor growth, from T1 (incidental) to T4 (invasion of neighboring organs).

> **Key points – epidemiology and pathophysiology**
>
> - Prostate cancer is likely soon to become the most common cause of cancer death in men.
> - Age is the greatest risk factor, but race, family history and intake of animal fats also have an impact.
> - Most prostate cancers are adenocarcinomas arising in the peripheral zone.
> - Prostate cancers are graded according to the Gleason system.

those that will definitely progress to clinical disease. Studies of incidental carcinomas diagnosed after TURP suggest that the median time to progression for T1b (high-volume, moderately or poorly differentiated) tumors is 4.75 years, compared with 13.5 years for T1a (low-volume, well-differentiated) tumors (Figure 1.10). Thus, elderly men with T1a tumors are more appropriately managed by active surveillance alone, while younger men with T1b disease may be

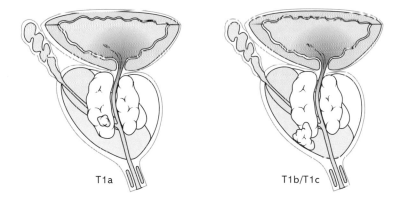

T1a   T1b/T1c

Figure 1.10 Incidental carcinoma of the prostate is unsuspected cancer diagnosed at TURP. T1a cancers are small, well-differentiated lesions involving less than 5% of resected tissue. T1b cancers are larger, involve more than 5% of the resected chippings and are less well-differentiated. T1c cancers detected by PSA testing are usually greater than 0.5 cm³ in volume and moderately well-differentiated.

considered for more aggressive, potentially curative therapy, such as radical prostatectomy or external-beam radiotherapy. Brachytherapy cannot be administered to men who have previously undergone TURP, because the radioactive seeds are not satisfactorily retained.

Key references

Bishop MC. Trends in prostate cancer mortality in England, Wales, and the USA. *Lancet Oncol* 2000;1:14.

Brawley OW, Barnes S, Parnes H. The future of prostate cancer prevention. *Ann N Y Acad Sci* 2001;952:145–52.

Brawley OW. Prostate carcinoma incidence and patient mortality. The effects of screening and early detection. *Cancer* 1997;80:1857–63.

Brooks JD, Metter EJ, Chan DW et al. Plasma selenium level before diagnosis and the risk of prostate cancer development. *J Urol* 2001;166:2034–8.

Carter BS, Bova S, Beaty TH et al. Hereditary prostate cancer: epidemiology and clinical features. *J Urol* 1993;150:797–802.

Chen C. Risk of prostate cancer in relation to polymorphisms of metabolic genes. *Epidemiol Rev* 2001;23:30–5.

Dennis LK, Resnick MI. Analysis of recent trends in prostate cancer incidence and mortality. *Prostate* 2000;42:247–52.

Fleshner NE. Vitamin E and prostate cancer. *Urol Clin North Am* 2002;29: 107–13.

Giovannucci E, Rimm EB, Liu Y et al. A prospective study of tomato products, lycopene, and prostate cancer risk. *J Natl Cancer Inst* 2002;94:391–8.

Gupta S, Mukhtar H. Green tea and prostate cancer. *Urol Clin North Am* 2002;29:49–57.

Krongrad A, Lai H, Lamm SH, Lai S. Mortality in prostate cancer. *J Urol* 1996;156:1084–91.

Lu-Yao GL, Greenberg ER. Changes in prostate cancer incidence and treatment in USA. *Lancet* 1994;343: 251–4.

Miller EC, Giovannucci E, Erdman JW Jr et al. Tomato products, lycopene, and prostate cancer risk. *Urol Clin North Am* 2002;29:83–93.

Montironi R, Mazzucchelli R, Scarpelli M. Precancerous lesions and conditions of the prostate: from morphological and biological characterization to chemoprevention. *Ann N Y Acad Sci* 2002;963:169–84.

Moyad MA. Lifestyle/dietary supplement partial androgen suppression and/or estrogen manipulation. A novel PSA reducer and preventive/treatment option for prostate cancer? *Urol Clin North Am* 2002;29:115–24.

Nelson MA, Reid M, Duffield-Lillico AJ, Marshall JR. Prostate cancer and selenium. *Urol Clin North Am* 2002; 29:67–70.

Nelson PS, Brawer MK. Chemoprevention of prostatic carcinoma. *Urology Int* 1997;4:7–9.

Nelson PS, Gleason TP, Brawer MK. Chemoprevention for prostatic intraepithelial neoplasia. *Eur Urol* 1996;30:269–78.

Parker SL, Tong T, Bolden S, Wingo PA. Cancer statistics, 1996. *CA Cancer J Clin* 1996;46:5–27.

Quinn M, Babb P. Patterns and trends in prostate cancer incidence, survival, prevalence and mortality. Part I: international comparisons. *BJU Int* 2002;90:162–73.

Roberts R, Jacobsen S, Kalusic SK et al. Recent declines in prostate cancer incidence and mortality. *J Urol* 1998;159:123A.

Rooney C, Beral V, Maconochie N et al. Case-control study of prostatic cancer in employees of the United Kingdom Atomic Energy Authority. *BMJ* 1993;307:1391–7.

Ross RK, Bernstain L, Lobo RA et al. 5 alpha-reductase activity and risk of prostate cancer among Japanese and US white and black males. *Lancet* 1992;339: 887–9.

Sarma AV, Schottenfeld D. Prostate cancer incidence, mortality, and survival trends in the United States: 1981-2001. *Semin Urol Oncol* 2002;20:3–9.

Sobin LH, Wittekind Ch, eds. *TNM classification of malignant tumours*, 5th edn. New York: Wiley–Liss, 1997.

Stanford JL, Stephenson RA, Coyle LM et al. *Prostate Cancer Trends 1973–1995, SEER Program, National Cancer Institute.* NIH Pub. No. 99–4543. Bethesda, MD, 1999.

Stephenson RA. Prostate cancer trends in the era of prostate-specific antigen. An update of incidence, mortality, and clinical factors from the SEER database. *Urol Clin North Am* 2002;29:173–81.

Thompson I, Goodman PJ, Tangen CM et al. The influence of finasteride on the development of prostate cancer. *N Engl J Med* 2003; 349:215–24.

The past decade has seen a significant downward shift in the stage of presentation of prostate cancer in most countries. Traditionally, most men with clinically significant disease presented with a combination of weight loss, bone pain, lethargy and bladder outflow obstruction, attributable to locally advanced or metastatic disease. Increasingly, however, the disease is being diagnosed in younger, asymptomatic patients, with much less advanced disease. This earlier presentation of prostate cancer has posed difficult dilemmas concerning management for clinicians and patients, and the increasing life expectancy of patients (Table 2.1) underscores the need for effective, evidence-based diagnosis and treatment regimens.

Diagnosis from clinical symptoms

Patients with prostate cancer may present with a variety of symptoms (Table 2.2). These principally consist of:

- symptoms of bladder outflow obstruction (frequency, hesitancy and poor flow), although much more commonly this is due to benign disease

TABLE 2.1

Survival statistics for US males with prostate cancer

Baseline Age	Probability of survival (%)			
	5 years	10 years	15 years	20 years
50	96	90	82	71
55	94	85	74	60
60	91	79	64	46
65	87	70	50	29
70	81	58	34	15
75	72	42	18	5

Source: *Vital Statistics of the United States*, 1989 US Life Tables, US National Center for Health Statistics

TABLE 2.2

Presenting symptoms of localized prostate cancer

Local disease	Locally invasive disease
• Asymptomatic	• Hematuria
• Elevated PSA	• Dysuria
• Weak stream	• Perineal and suprapubic pain
• Hesitancy	• Impotence
• Sensation of incomplete emptying	• Incontinence
• Frequency	• Loin pain or anuria resulting from obstruction of the ureters
• Urgency	• Symptoms of renal failure
• Urge incontinence	• Hemospermia
• Urinary tract infection	• Rectal symptoms including tenesmus

- symptoms resulting from local extension of the tumor, such as hematuria or pain due to hydronephrosis secondary to obstruction of the ureters
- symptoms resulting from distant metastases, such as low back pain, spinal cord compression, bone pain, anemia or weight loss.

Bladder outflow obstruction symptoms may be attributable either to prostate cancer itself, particularly if the disease is locally advanced, or, more commonly, to concomitant BPH. Symptoms may be classified as obstructive or irritative. Obstructive symptoms, which include a weak urine stream, hesitancy and incomplete emptying, are a direct result of compression of the urethra by the tumor. Irritative symptoms are due to detrusor instability secondary to obstruction; such symptoms include urinary frequency and urgency (an inability to postpone urination). Irritative symptoms in patients with prostate cancer may also occur as a result of invasion by the tumor of the bladder trigone and pelvic nerves.

23

The severity of symptoms can be assessed by means of the International Prostate Symptom Score (IPSS). This consists of eight questions; seven relate to specific symptoms, and one addresses the impact of symptoms on the patient's quality of life (Figure 2.1).

Bladder outflow obstruction due to either BPH or prostate cancer can lead to complications such as recurrent urinary tract infections, which may in turn produce further symptoms such as frequency, dysuria or hematuria. Acute or chronic urinary retention may also develop as a result of either prostate cancer or associated BPH.

Symptoms of locally invasive prostate cancer. In addition to symptoms of bladder outflow obstruction, local invasion can produce a variety of symptoms.

- Hematuria and dysuria may result from direct invasion of the prostatic urethra, while invasion of the urethral sphincter or surgery itself may cause urinary incontinence. It is important to exclude the possibility that incontinence is a result of chronic urinary retention with overflow, which may be amenable to treatment with procedures such as TURP.
- Extension of the tumor beyond the prostatic capsule may affect the neurovascular bundles that lie adjacent to the prostate; this may lead to erectile dysfunction (Figure 2.2). Similarly, involvement of the perineal or suprapubic nerves can lead to pain, and thus the possibility of prostate cancer should be considered in the investigation of prostatitis-like symptoms.
- Locally advanced disease may impinge on the distal rectum and lead to symptoms such as constipation, tenesmus and rectal bleeding.
- Invasion of the seminal vesicles may occasionally result in hemospermia, but this is not a common symptom in prostate cancer.

Symptoms of metastatic disease. Worldwide, many men with prostate cancer still present with metastatic disease. The most common presenting symptoms are shown in Table 2.3. Pain resulting from bony metastases, particularly in the pelvis and lumbar spine, is the major

	Not at all	1 time in 5	Less than half the time	Less than the time	About half the time	More than half the time	Almost always	Patient score
1 Incomplete emptying Over the past month, how often have you had a sensation of not emptying your bladder completely after you finished urinating?	0	1	2	3	4	5		
2 Frequency Over the past month, how often have you had to urinate again less than 2 hours after you finished urinating?	0	1	2	3	4	5		
3 Intermittency Over the past month, how often have you found you stopped and started again several times when you urinated?	0	1	2	3	4	5		
4 Urgency Over the past month, how often have you found it difficult to postpone urination?	0	1	2	3	4	5		
5 Weak stream Over the past month, how often have you had a weak urinary stream?	0	1	2	3	4	5		
6 Straining Over the past month, how often have you had to push or strain to begin urination?	0	1	2	3	4	5		
7 Nocturia Over the past month, how many times did you most typically get up to urinate from the time you went to bed at night until the time you got up in the morning?	0	1	2	3	4	5+		
Total IPSS								

	Delighted	Pleased	Mostly satisfied	Mixed	Mostly dissatisfied	Unhappy	Terrible
Quality of life due to urinary symptoms If you were to spend the rest of your life with your urinary condition the way it is now, how would you feel about that?	0	1	2	3	4	5	6

Figure 2.1 The severity of urinary symptoms can be assessed with the International Prostate Symptom Score (IPSS): < 8, mild; 8–20, moderate; > 20, severe.

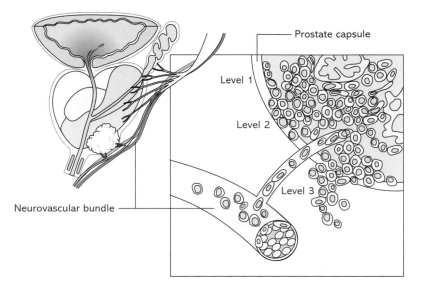

Figure 2.2 Prostate cancer penetrating the prostatic capsule and involving the neurovascular bundle.

symptom; thus, the sudden onset of progressive low back or pelvic pain is an important diagnostic feature of metastatic prostate cancer. Pathological fractures may also occur, particularly affecting the neck of

TABLE 2.3

Presenting symptoms of metastatic prostate cancer

Distant metastases

- Bone pain or sciatica
- Paraplegia secondary to spinal cord compression
- Lymph node enlargement
- Loin pain or anuria due to obstruction of the ureters by lymph nodes

Widespread metastases

- Lethargy (e.g. due to anemia or uremia)
- Weight loss and cachexia
- Cutaneous and bowel hemorrhage (unusual)

the femur. Metastases within the vertebrae, sometimes leading to spinal cord compression, are not uncommon and may produce backache or neurological symptoms in up to 12% of affected patients.

Metastasis into the lymph nodes may result in lymph node enlargement. Intra-abdominal lymph node metastasis usually begins in the obturator and internal iliac nodes, spreads to the iliac nodes and beyond, and may, with local tumors, result in obstruction of the ureters. In advanced disease, lymphatic involvement may extend to the thoracic, cervical, inguinal and axillary nodes. Lymph node metastases may produce a number of symptoms, including palpable swellings, loin pain or anuria due to obstruction of the ureters, and swelling of the lower limbs as a result of lymphedema.

Systemic metastases in the liver, lungs or elsewhere may produce non-specific symptoms, such as lethargy resulting from anemia or uremia, weight loss and cachexia.

Incidental diagnosis of prostate cancer

Prostate cancer may still present as an 'incidental' finding after TURP (Figure 2.3); nowadays < 10% of men undergoing TURP for BPH are found to have microscopic foci of prostate cancer. In approximately two-thirds of cases, well-differentiated tumors are present in less than 5% of the resected chips; this is referred to as stage T1a disease. In the remaining cases, which are classified as stage T1b disease, tumors are less well-differentiated (Gleason score > 4), and more than 5% of the resected tissue may be involved.

The diagnosis of prostate cancer after TURP may be subject to sampling errors, as resected chips are mainly derived from the transition zone, and fewer than 30% of prostate cancers arise in this region. Thus, a tumor that is localized to the transition zone may have been completely excised during TURP, whereas significant amounts of multifocal or locally invasive tumors are still present in the residual peripheral prostatic tissue after the operation (Figure 2.3). This may present difficulties in assessing the prognosis for an individual patient, and in selecting the optimal treatment modality. PSA measurement and transrectal biopsy of the residual prostate tissue often help to clarify the position.

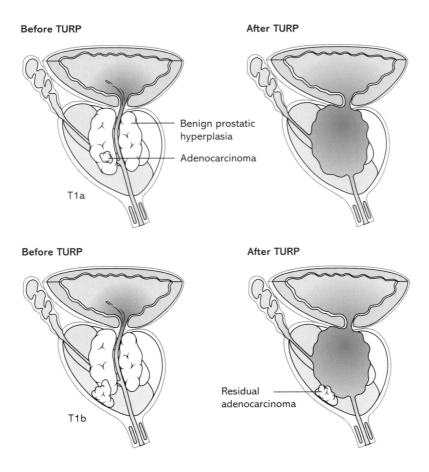

Before TURP

After TURP

Benign prostatic
hyperplasia

Adenocarcinoma

T1a

Before TURP

After TURP

Residual
adenocarcinoma

T1b

Figure 2.3 Prostate cancer is found in resected chips of prostate tissue obtained during TURP in up to 10% of cases. About two thirds of these are well-differentiated T1a lesions involving less than 5% of the chips. The remaining lesions are larger volume, less well differentiated T1b cancers. A number of potential sampling errors are inherent in the diagnosis of prostate cancer at TURP. T1a tumors that are confined to the transition zone may be completely excised, whereas significant amounts of T1b tumors may remain after the procedure.

Early detection of prostate cancer

In general, the earlier prostate cancer is detected, the better the outlook for the patient in terms of cure or arresting cancer progression. Most patients in whom prostate cancer is suspected are identified on the basis of abnormal findings on digital rectal examination (DRE) or, more commonly now, by raised PSA levels. An increasing majority of patients present simply with an isolated increase in PSA value.

Digital rectal examination is the simplest, safest and most cost-effective means of detecting prostate cancer, provided that the tumor is posteriorly situated and is sufficiently large to be palpable. The test can be performed with the patient either in the left lateral position or standing and leaning forwards; with either approach only the posterior portion of the gland is palpable (Figure 2.4). In addition to providing information on the size of the prostate, DRE can reveal a number of features that may indicate prostate cancer (Table 2.4). However, only around one-third of suspect prostatic nodules are actually confirmed as malignant when analysed histologically after transrectal biopsy (Table 2.5).

Prostate-specific antigen is a glycoprotein responsible for liquefying semen. Approximately 20% of men with PSA levels above the normal

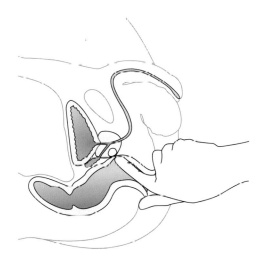

Figure 2.4 DRE is an essential clinical test in the detection and diagnosis of prostate cancer.

TABLE 2.4

DRE findings that may indicate prostate cancer

- Asymmetry of the gland
- A nodule within one lobe of the gland
- Induration of part or all of the prostate
- Lack of mobility due to adhesion to surrounding tissue
- Palpable seminal vesicles

TABLE 2.5

Causes of false-positive diagnoses of prostate cancer on DRE

- Benign prostatic hyperplasia
- Prostatic calculi
- Prostatitis (particularly granulomatous prostatitis)
- Ejaculatory duct abnormalities
- Seminal vesicle abnormalities
- Rectal mucosal polyp or tumor

range (≥ 4 ng/mL) have prostate cancer, and the risk increases to more than 60% in men with PSA levels above 10 ng/mL (Figure 2.5). PSA measurement is the most effective single screening test for early detection of prostate cancer; in fact, it can detect more than twice as many prostate cancers as DRE. However, the predictive value is increased further if the measurement is combined, as it always should be, with DRE. PSA determinations may also be useful in the staging of prostate cancer and evaluating the response to therapy (see Chapter 3).

Nevertheless, PSA is by no means perfect, as many men with mildly elevated PSA values do not have prostate cancer. As a result, several different concepts have been developed over the past few years to improve the clinical value of the test in detecting early prostate cancer. These so-called PSA derivatives include PSA density, PSA velocity, age-specific reference ranges and differential assay of the different molecular forms of serum PSA.

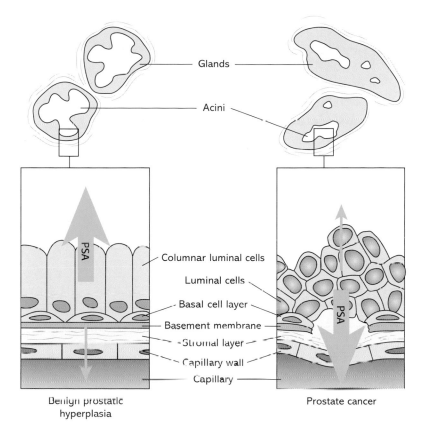

Figure 2.5 Normally, there are significant tissue barriers between the lumen of the prostate gland and the capillary bed. In prostatic diseases, especially cancer, these barriers are compromised, and serum PSA values rise.

- PSA density correlates the serum PSA concentration with the volume of the prostate gland.
- PSA velocity refers to the change in PSA with time, usually over 1 or 2 years.
- The age-specific reference ranges are based on the fact that the serum PSA concentration increases with advancing age. As a result, the reference range is corrected for the patient's age.
- PSA exists in the serum in several molecular forms; most of it is bound to protein, some is unbound, or 'free'. Recent data show that patients with BPH only have a higher amount of free PSA, and men

31

with prostate cancer appear to have a greater amount of PSA that is complexed to α_1-antichymotrypsin. Measuring the concentration of these different molecular forms in the serum is currently the most clinically useful way to distinguish men who have BPH only from patients with early prostate cancer. The currently accepted cut-off point of free:total PSA is 0.15. Patients with ratios below this should be considered for further investigation, including transrectal prostatic biopsies.

However, the first three PSA derivatives are of limited clinical impact. Figure 2.6 demonstrates the sampling bias of PSA density. PSA velocity is problematic, too, owing to significant biological variation. Finally, Figure 2.7 shows the problems with an age-specific cut-off as opposed to a standard cut-off for all ages – too many cancers are missed in older men (in whom the prevalence is greater).

All of these concepts are attempts to enhance the utility of PSA with regard to detecting early prostate cancer at a curable stage and to reduce the number of negative transrectal biopsies. In practical terms, only the free:total PSA ratio is clinically useful, since it can help the physician and patient decide whether and when to proceed to a transrectal biopsy.

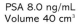 PSA 8.0 ng/mL
Volume 40 cm³

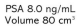 PSA 8.0 ng/mL
Volume 80 cm³

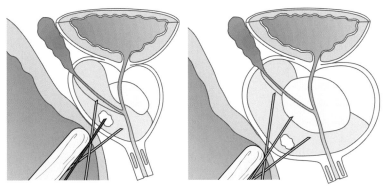

Figure 2.6 Biopsies taken from a larger prostate with a lower PSA density are less likely to sample the cancer than those taken from a smaller prostate with a higher PSA density.

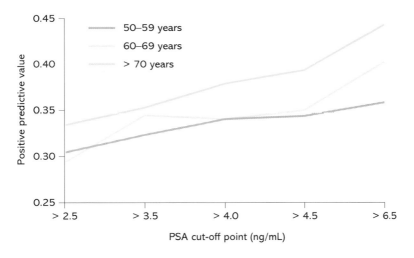

Figure 2.7 Raising the PSA cut-off point in older men increases the positive predictive value, but reduces the overall detection rate.

Screening for prostate cancer. The value of screening asymptomatic men for prostate cancer is controversial (Table 2.6). As described in Chapter 1, there is a great discrepancy between the incidence of clinically significant disease and the prevalence of microscopic disease, and identification of those patients in whom disease progression is probable remains inexact. Thus, early detection has not yet been shown to lead to improved survival among patients with clinical disease, although the recent reduction in prostate cancer mortality may point to efficacy of early detection and treatment. Furthermore, several studies on stored sera from men who subsequently developed prostate cancer have shown that PSA testing is highly discriminatory between these men and age-matched controls. Moreover, those patients identified as having prostate cancer on screening usually harbor clinically significant, potentially life-threatening tumors. Clearly, early detection could potentially lead to benefits in terms of reduced morbidity and hence improved quality of life, and prolonged survival. Conversely, however, older men may not derive the same benefits as younger men, as significant disease progression is less likely within their lifetime. It is hoped that ongoing, prospective, randomized studies of screening in the USA and in Europe will clarify the situation. In the meantime, the

TABLE 2.6

Screening for prostate cancer

Pros

- Simple tests available (PSA and DRE)
- Detects early, potentially curable lesions
- Reassures those who are screened as negative
- May reduce prostate cancer morbidity and mortality

Cons

- More likely to detect slow-growing tumors
- Unproven efficacy in reducing mortality
- Some cancers detected may never present clinically
- False-positive findings cause anxiety
- Expensive, uncomfortable and time-consuming
- Biopsy guided by TRUS carries a 2% risk of serious infective complications

family physician has an important role in assessing the likely benefits and risks for individual patients according to their age and life expectancy; appropriate counseling of the patient and his immediate family is an essential element of this process.

Key points – clinical presentation

- Increasingly, prostate cancer is being diagnosed on the basis of increased PSA values.
- Screening of asymptomatic men by PSA tests is controversial.
- Transrectal ultrasound-guided biopsies are needed to confirm the diagnosis.
- More advanced disease can present with symptoms of bladder outflow obstruction.
- Bone metastases may cause bone pain or pathological fracture.

Key references

Benson MC, Whang IS, Panteuck A et al. Prostate specific antigen density: a means of distinguishing between benign prostatic hypertrophy and prostate cancer. *J Urol* 1992;147: 815–16.

Brawer MK. Clinical usefulness of assays for complexed prostate-specific antigen. *Urol Clin N Am* 2002;29: 193–203.

Brawer MK, Meyer GE, Letran JL et al. Measurement of complexed PSA improves specificity for early detection of prostate cancer. *Urology* 1998;52:379–83.

Brawley OW. Prostate carcinoma incidence and patient mortality: the effects of screening and early detection. *Cancer* 1997;80:1857–63.

Carter BH, Pearson JD, Metter J et al. Longitudinal evaluation of prostate specific antigen levels in men with and without prostate cancer. *JAMA* 1993;267:2215–20.

Catalona WJ, Partin AW, Slawin KM et al. Use of the percentage of free prostate-specific antigen to enhance differentiation of prostate cancer from benign prostatic disease: a prospective multicenter clinical trial. *JAMA* 1998;279:1542–7.

Christensson A, Bjork T, Nilsson O et al. Serum prostate specific antigen complexed to alpha-1-antichymotrypsin as an indicator of prostate cancer. *J Urol* 1993;150: 100–5.

de Koning HJ, Auvinen A, Berenguer Sanchez A et al. Large-scale randomized prostate cancer screening trials: program performances in the European Randomized Screening for Prostate Cancer trial and the Prostate, Lung, Colorectal and Ovary cancer trial. *Int J Cancer* 2002;97:237–44.

de Koning HJ, Liem MK, Baan CA et al. Prostate cancer mortality reduction by screening: power and time frame with complete enrollment in the European Randomised Screening for Prostate Cancer (ERSPC) trial. *Int J Cancer* 2002;98: 268–73.

Djavan B, Remzi M, Schulman CC et al. Repeat prostate biopsy: who, how and when? A review. *Eur Urol* 2002,42:93–103.

Gleason DF, Mellinger GT. Prediction of prognosis for prostatic adenocarcinoma by combined histological grading and clinical staging. 1974. *J Urol* 2002;167(2 pt 2):953–8; discussion 959.

Kirby RS, Kirby MG, Feneley MR et al. Screening for carcinoma of the prostate: a GP based study. *Br J Urol* 1994;74:64–71.

Neal DE, Donovan JL. Prostate cancer: to screen or not to screen? *Lancet Oncol* 2000;1:17–24.

Nixon RG, Brawer MK. Enhancing the specificity of prostate-specific antigen: an overview of PSA density, PSA velocity and age-specific PSA reference ranges. *Br J Urol* 1997; 79:61–7.

Oesterling JE, Jacobsen SJ, Chute CG et al. Serum prostate-specific antigen in a community-based population of healthy men. *JAMA* 1993;270:860–4.

Oesterling JE, Jacobsen SJ, Chute CG et al. The establishment of age-specific reference ranges for prostate-specific antigen. *J Urol* 1993;149: 510A.

Okihara K, Cheli CD, Partin AW et al. Comparative analysis of prostate specific antigen, free prostate specific antigen and their ratio in detecting prostate cancer. *J Urol* 2002;167:2017–23 (discussion 2023–24).

Okihara K, Cheli CD, Partin AW et al. Comparative analysis of complexed prostate specific antigen, free prostate specific antigen and their ratio in detecting prostate cancer. *J Urol* 2002;167:2017–23.

Parkes C, Wald NJ, Murphy P et al. Prospective observational study to assess value of PSA as screening test for prostate cancer. *BMJ* 1995; 311:1340–3.

Partin AW, Brawer MK, Subong ENP et al. Prospective evaluation of percent free-PSA and complexed-PSA for early detection of prostate cancer. *Prostate Cancer Prostatic Diseases* 1998;1:197–203.

Schröder FH, Wildhagen MF. Screening for prostate cancer: evidence and perspectives. *BJU Int.* 2001;88:811–7.

Singh Kalsi G. Demand for prostate specific antigen testing in primary care. Can the demand for PSA testing in primary care be managed? *BMJ* 2002;324:547.

Van Cangh PJ, Nayer PD, Sauvage P. Free to total PSA ratio is superior to total PSA in differentiating BPH from prostate cancer. *Prostate* 1996;7: 30–4.

Van Der Cruijsen-Koeter IW, Wildhagen MF, De Koning HJ, Schroder FH. The value of current diagnostic tests in prostate cancer screening. *BJU Int* 2001;88:458–66.

Woodrum DL, Brawer MK, Partin AW et al. Interpretation of free prostate-specific antigen clinical research studies for the detection of prostate cancer. *J Urol* 1998;159: 5–12.

Accurate grading and staging of prostate cancer, particularly distinguishing between Gleason grades and between localized and extensive disease, is important for selection of the best treatment option. Although developments in imaging techniques have led to more accurate staging than can be achieved with DRE or PSA testing alone, both under- and overstaging are still common clinical problems. Thus, a need remains not only for improved staging techniques, but also for better prognostic indicators.

Staging of localized disease

Staging of localized disease relies primarily on the following techniques:

- DRE
- PSA measurement
- transrectal ultrasonography (TRUS) and ultrasound-guided biopsy
- computerized tomography (CT) scanning
- magnetic resonance imaging (MRI)
- a combination of DRE, PSA and biopsy information.

Digital rectal examination. The accuracy of DRE in diagnosing and staging prostate cancer is approximately 30–50%; underestimation is common because small and anteriorly located tumors are generally impalpable, and false-positive findings may occur in patients with conditions such as BPH or prostatitis. The technique can, however, detect a number of significant cancers when PSA is still within the normal range (< 4.0 ng/mL) and provide useful, if imprecise, information about the local stage of the disease (Table 3.1).

Prostate-specific antigen determination. Within groups of patients, there is a reasonable correlation between PSA levels and the pathological stage (and, to a lesser extent, the clinical stage) of prostate cancer. The correlation is poorer, however, in individual patients because of the

TABLE 3.1

Clinical staging of localized prostate cancer by DRE

Tumor stage	DRE findings
T2a	Peripheral, firm nodule; no apparent distortion of capsule
T2b	Hard, more irregular; unilateral enlargement may be present
T3	Irregular distortion; prostate remains mobile; seminal vesicles may be palpable
T4	Gross enlargement; hard and irregular; prostate immobile owing to adhesion to surrounding tissues

considerable overlap between the PSA ranges associated with different stages. PSA levels above 10–20 ng/mL are often indicative of tumor extension beyond the prostatic capsule, while levels above 40 ng/mL suggest the presence of bony or soft tissue metastases.

Although the serum PSA concentration alone may not be a precise indicator of stage on an individual basis, it can sometimes be used to eliminate some staging investigations. It appears that men who present with newly diagnosed, well or moderately well differentiated prostate cancer, no skeletal symptoms and a serum PSA value less than or equal to 10 ng/mL may not always need a staging radionuclide bone scan. For these individuals, the probability of having skeletal metastases approaches zero. Many clinicians, however, still like to use this test as a baseline investigation because it may identify 'hot spots' due to conditions such as degenerative osteoarthritis that may cause confusion later, if and when the PSA level starts to rise. A negative scan also serves to reassure the patients that the skeleton is uninvolved.

It is also now clear that the combination of serum PSA concentration, tumor grade from the biopsy specimens and the local clinical stage from the DRE can be used to estimate the clinical stage. For instance, a man with a clinical stage T2a prostate cancer, a primary Gleason grade 3 and a serum PSA of 6 ng/mL probably does not need to undergo a staging bilateral pelvic lymphadenectomy; the probability of this individual having positive pelvic lymph nodes approaches zero. The relationship between tumor grade, clinical stage and PSA value in terms of predicting tumor curability has been computed and summarized in Partin's tables (Figure 3.1). These tables are particularly helpful when discussing treatment options and the probability of extraprostatic extension and consequently the chances of surgical cure.

Figure 3.2 demonstrates how the preoperative serum PSA predicts clinical outcome (i.e. the risk of biochemical recurrence).

Transrectal ultrasonography (TRUS). Accurate images of the prostate can be obtained by TRUS, in which an ultrasound probe is introduced into the rectum to lie adjacent to the prostate (Figure 3.3). The normal prostate is well defined and symmetrical, and surrounded by a discrete capsule. The transition zone is visible as a hypoechoic area. In patients with prostate cancer, however, a number of ultrasonographic abnormalities may be present, including:
- abnormal echo patterns (usually hypoechoic)
- loss of differentiation between central and peripheral zones
- asymmetry of size or shape
- capsular distortion.

Approximately two thirds of prostate tumors are hypoechoic. Hypoechoic images may result from other causes, however, so the

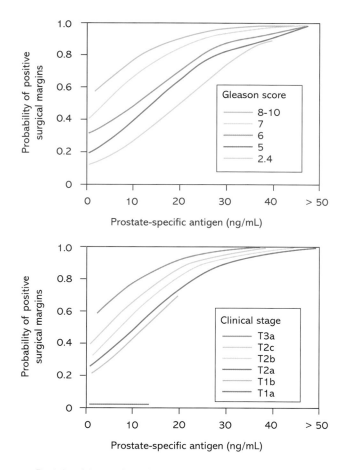

Figure 3.1 Partin's tables are based on the retrospective analysis of several thousand patients undergoing radical prostatectomy. They relate PSA, tumor grade and clinical stage to the probability of extraprostatic extension.

specificity of this finding for prostate cancer is only 20–25%. TRUS can sometimes be useful to estimate the extent of extraprostatic extension and seminal vesicle involvement (generally a contraindication for radical prostatectomy), but biopsy confirmation is usually required.

By far the most valuable role for TRUS is in directing the biopsy of prostate tumors. It is more accurate and convenient than digital guidance as the biopsy needle can be guided through a port incorporated in the ultrasound probe and its position visualized directly.

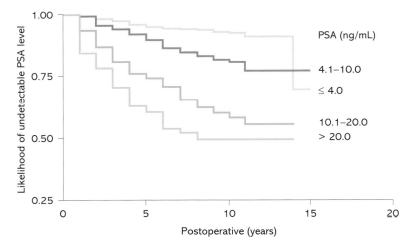

Figure 3.2 Kaplan–Meier actuarial likelihood of prostate-specific antigen recurrence after radical prostatectomy by preoperative serum PSA levels.

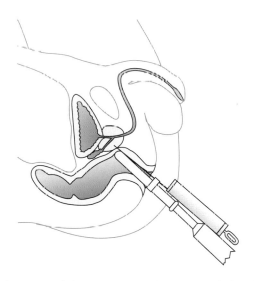

Figure 3.3 TRUS imaging of the prostate is an important technique in diagnosis and staging of prostate cancer. An ultrasound probe is introduced into the rectum to lie adjacent to the prostate. Under antibiotic cover and ultrasound control, multiple prostatic biopsies may be taken with an automatic biopsy gun.

Most prostatic biopsies are now performed by this technique. Antibiotic treatment, usually with a quinolone, is given before and after the procedure to reduce the risk of infection, which is currently estimated at around 2%. Usually six to eight, but sometimes as many as twelve, TRUS-guided biopsies are now routinely performed on an outpatient basis, preferably after infiltration with local anesthesia. The percentage of each biopsy core involved and the overall number of positive biopsy specimens provide a useful estimate of tumor volume (Figure 3.4). In high-risk cases (PSA > 20 ng/mL or Gleason score > 7), additional lateral capsular and seminal vesicle biopsies can be taken with minimal extra morbidity to confirm or exclude extraprostatic extension.

MRI and CT scanning can be used to examine the internal structure of the prostate. These techniques have not been clearly shown to be more effective than TRUS in staging localized prostate cancer, and there is some evidence that TRUS with additional biopsies is in fact more accurate in staging more advanced (T2 and T3) disease. At

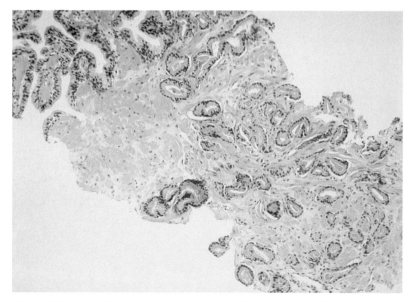

Figure 3.4 A prostatic biopsy core positive for adenocarcinoma (Gleason grades 3 and 4, Gleason score 7).

present, therefore, TRUS remains the 'gold standard' imaging technique for staging localized prostate cancer, though ever-improving endorectal MRI technology and gadolinium enhancement can sometimes be helpful in confirming suspected seminal-vesicle or lymph-node involvement.

Staging of metastatic disease

Staging of metastatic disease involves assessing the extent of bone and soft tissue involvement. The principal techniques used are a chest X-ray, radionuclide bone scanning, and CT and MRI scanning.

Radionuclide bone scanning is usually performed as a baseline assessment at the time of the initial diagnosis of prostate cancer (Figure 3.5). If the PSA value is < 10 ng/mL and Gleason score is > 8, it may be permissible to omit this test as it is rarely positive in these circumstances. The use of this technique in routine follow-up has declined as PSA measurements have been shown to be the most accurate and cost-effective means of monitoring bony metastases.

CT scanning of the abdomen and pelvis may be used in cases in which treatment decisions depend on the presence and degree of lymph node involvement. Small volume and microscopic metastases (< 2 cm) are

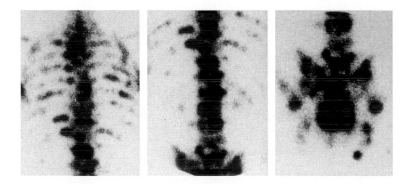

Figure 3.5 A radionuclide bone scan showing multiple bony metastases resulting from disseminated prostate cancer.

not usually detectable by this technique, and thus the accuracy of CT scanning is only approximately 40–50%. CT scanning may also be employed occasionally to guide skinny needle aspiration of enlarged lymph nodes for cytological analysis to aid diagnosis.

MRI scanning can also be used to identify metastatic disease affecting the regional lymph nodes. However, in most scanners the technique does not permit guided skinny needle aspiration, and it is not usually indicated if the PSA is below 10 ng/mL. MRI scanning may also be useful in clarifying the nature of any abnormality in equivocal bone scans.

Immunoscintigraphy using radioactive antibodies directed against prostate-specific proteins has proved inadequate for clinical use in its present form owing to lack of specificity and sensitivity.

Approach to staging and management

An approach to the diagnosis, staging and management of localized prostate cancer is outlined in Figure 3.6.

Key points – staging prostate cancer

- Prostate cancer is usually diagnosed on the basis of transrectal ultrasound-guided biopsies under antibiotic cover and local anesthesia.
- The Gleason score of these biopsies, the clinical stage on DRE and the presenting PSA value provide an estimate of the risk of extraprostatic extension.
- MRI and CT scanning can provide information about local staging.
- Bone scanning identifies bone metastases, but the probability these are present is low when PSA values are < 10 ng/mL.

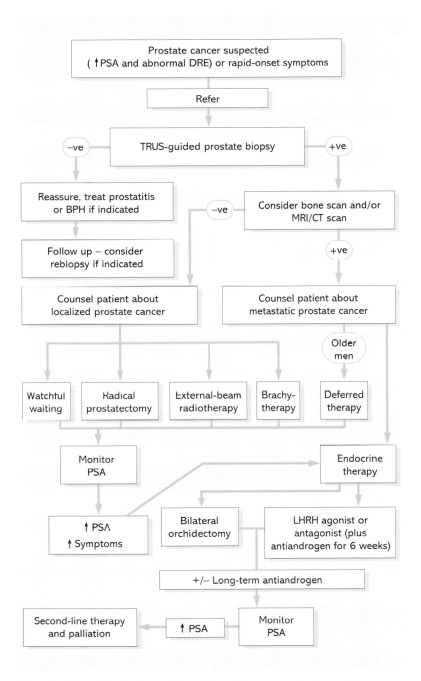

Figure 3.6 Algorithm for diagnosis, staging and management of prostate cancer.

Key references

Bernstein MR, Wein AJ, Siegelman ES et al. Lack of correlation of clinical and pathologic staging of capsular involvement in prostate cancer using endorectal coil magnetic resonance imaging. *J Pelvic Surg* 1999;5:203–7.

Brawer MK, Meyer GE. Prostate cancer: staging and prognostic markers. In: A Belldegrun, Kirby RS, Newling DWW, eds. *New Perspectives in Prostate Cancer*. 2nd edn. Oxford: Isis Medical Media, 2000.

Brawer MK. Radiation therapy failure in prostate cancer patients: risk factors and methods of detection. *Rev Urol* 2002;4:suppl 2:S2–S11.

Davis M, Sofer M, Kim SS, Soloway MS. The procedure of transrectal ultrasound guided biopsy of the prostate: a survey of patient preparation and biopsy technique. *J Urol* 2002;167:566–70.

Gleason DF. Histologic grading in clinical staging of prostatic carcinoma. In: Tannenbaum M, ed. *Urologic pathology: the prostate*. Philadelphia: Lea & Febiger, 1977:171–98.

Han M, Partin AW. Nomograms for clinically localized prostate cancer. Part I: radical prostatectomy. *Semin Urol Oncol* 2002;20:123–30.

Makarov DV, Sanderson H, Partin AW, Epstein JI. Gleason score 7 prostate cancer on needle biopsy: is the prognostic difference in Gleason scores 4 + 3 and 3 + 4 independent of the number of involved cores? *J Urol* 2002;167:2440–2.

Miller PD, Eardley I, Kirby RS. Prostate specific antigen and bone scan correlation in staging and monitoring of prostate cancer. *Br J Urol* 1992;70:295–8.

Moul JW, Kane CJ, Malkowicz SB. The role of imaging studies and molecular markers for selecting candidates for radical prostatectomy. *Urol Clin North Am* 2001;28:459–72.

Narain V, Bianco FJ Jr, Grignon DJ et al. How accurately does prostate biopsy Gleason score predict pathologic findings and disease free survival? *Prostate* 2001;49:185–90.

Oesterling JE. Using prostate specific antigen to eliminate the staging radionuclide bone scan: significant economic implications. *Urol Clin N Am* 1993;20:705–12.

Ohori M, Swindle P. Nomograms and instruments for the initial prostate evaluation: the ability to estimate the likelihood of identifying prostate cancer. *Semin Urol Oncol* 2002;20:116–22.

Partin AW, Natlan MW, Subong ENP. Combination of prostate specific antigen, clinical stage and Gleason score to predict pathological stage of localized prostate cancer. *JAMA* 1997;277:1445–51.

Scherr DS, Eastham J, Ohori M, Scardino PT. Prostate biopsy techniques and indications: when, where, and how? *Semin Urol Oncol* 2002;20:18–31.

Taneja SS, Hsu EI, Cheli CD et al. Complexed prostate-specific antigen as a staging tool: results based on a multicenter prospective evaluation of complexed prostate-specific antigen in cancer diagnosis. *Urology* 2002;60(4 suppl 1):10–7.

The aim of treatment in patients with localized prostate cancer is usually cure – whether eliminating the tumor or preventing death from prostate cancer (as opposed to death with prostate cancer), provided that the individual has a life expectancy of at least 10 years. As men with localized disease often do not experience significant disease-related morbidity for several years after diagnosis, and curative treatment itself may result in some morbidity, those with a shorter life expectancy are likely to benefit least from radical treatment. The available treatment options are listed in Table 4.1. Unfortunately, our current state of knowledge is such that it is not always possible to say which of these will produce the optimum outcome in an individual patient. In some cases a simple policy of active surveillance (watchful waiting) with the option of rebiopsy in due course may be the best option.

TABLE 4.1

Treatment options for localized prostate cancer

- Active surveillance (watchful waiting)
- Radiotherapy
    - external beam
    - conformal
- Brachytherapy
- Radical prostatectomy (retropubic, perineal or laparoscopic)
- Approaches under investigation
    - cryotherapy
    - laser therapy
    - high-intensity focused ultrasound
    - adjuvant treatment with antiandrogen

Prognostic indicators

One of the most helpful innovations for the future would be the development of more reliable prognostic indicators for prostate cancer. These would facilitate the selection of appropriate therapy, taking into account the likely future behavior of a given cancer. Traditionally, the best indicator is the Gleason score, but other molecular indicators promise to be valuable. For example, metastatic cancer can only develop and grow beyond a certain size if it acquires an adequate blood supply; this requires angiogenesis (the development of new blood vessels). Such angiogenic areas can now be assayed automatically and a mean vessel density score ascribed. Other molecular indicators of progression include the loss of cell adhesion molecules, such as E-cadherin, which is involved in cell-to-cell attachments and appears to be antimetastatic. Recently Sinha et al. have reported that anti-cathepsin B and stefin A may be useful new immunohistochemical markers. A number of other types of markers of malignant potential currently under intensive investigation are shown in Table 4.2.

Active surveillance

A policy of active surveillance (watchful waiting) may be appropriate in older patients with low-volume, well-differentiated tumors, particularly when other significant illnesses are also present. Patients should be

---

TABLE 4.2

Prostate markers of malignant potential

- Grade
- Clinical stage
- Pathological stage
- Tumor volume
- PSA
- DNA ploidy
- Nuclear morphometry
- Neovascularity
- Oncogenes
- Tumor suppressor genes
- Invasion markers (cathepsin, collagenase)
- Cell-adherence markers
- Basement membrane (collagen)
- Growth factors
- Growth factor receptors
- Others

counseled, reviewed and reassured, and PSA levels measured at regular intervals. This approach may also be appropriate for older patients with larger tumors, as long-term studies have suggested a low rate of metastasis in some of these individuals. In a recent meta-analysis, the development of metastatic disease during active surveillance was reported to be 2.1% per year in patients with well-differentiated tumors (Gleason scores 2–4), compared with 13.5% per year in patients with aggressive tumors (Gleason scores 7–10). Patients with low-grade tumors had a disease-specific survival rate of 87% after 10 years, compared with only 26% in patients with poorly differentiated tumors. However, if the PSA value shows evidence of sequential rise or the patient becomes concerned, rebiopsy and/or initiation of therapy should be considered after a thorough discussion of the issues, including a description of the probability of side effects of treatment, with the patient and his family.

Radical prostatectomy

Radical prostatectomy involves surgical removal of the entire prostate, the seminal vesicles and a variable amount of adjacent tissue (Figure 4.1). It is appropriate for men in whom it is believed the tumor can be removed completely by surgery, and who satisfy the criteria in Table 4.3. The procedure is most commonly performed via the retropubic route, though the perineal approach can also be used. The major advantage of radical prostatectomy is that it excises all prostatic tissue and provides precise histological information and definitive cure in patients in whom the tumor is specimen-confined. Thus, the patient's anxiety is relieved during the postoperative period; given that prostate cancer has a long natural history, this is an important consideration in terms of the patient's quality of life. Long-term studies have shown normal life expectancies in those with complete excision of specimen-confined disease and overall 15-year metastasis-free survival rates of up to 82%. Moreover, the procedure also offers definitive treatment of concomitant BPH. Principal adverse events associated with radical prostatectomy are persistent urinary incontinence (< 2–3%) and ED (> 50%), though the latter is age-related, tends to improve with time and can be minimized by nerve-sparing approaches and more recently

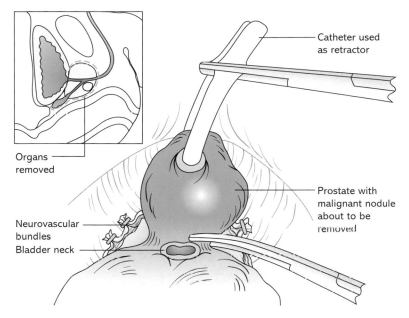

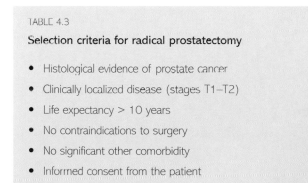

Figure 4.1 Radical prostatectomy. The entire prostate and attached seminal vesicles can be removed surgically and an anastomosis created between the bladder neck and the urethra.

by intraoperative nerve grafting. Moreover, ED after surgery can now be treated effectively (see Chapter 8). Table 4.4 summarizes the advantages and disadvantages of radical prostatectomy.

Recently laparoscopic radical prostatectomy has been described. It can be facilitated by robotic assistance. The results of the procedure

TABLE 4.3

Selection criteria for radical prostatectomy

- Histological evidence of prostate cancer
- Clinically localized disease (stages T1–T2)
- Life expectancy > 10 years
- No contraindications to surgery
- No significant other comorbidity
- Informed consent from the patient

TABLE 4.4

Advantages and disadvantages of radiotherapy, radical prostatectomy or brachytherapy in the treatment of localized prostate cancer

Radiotherapy

Advantages

- Potential cure
- Surgery avoided
- Outpatient therapy
- Enhanced by hormone ablation therapy

Disadvantages

- Prostate left in situ
- Difficulty assessing cure
- No definitive staging possible
- No benefit on concomitant BPH
- Patient anxiety during follow-up
- Unreliable PSA suppression
- Potential morbidity:
  - rectal injury (2–10%)
  - urinary incontinence (< 3%)
  - impotence (20–30%)
  - bladder damage (10–20%)
  - hematuria (5–10%)
- Surgery after radiotherapy not feasible

Radical prostatectomy

Advantages

- Cure if tumor pathologically confined
- Definitive staging possible
- Treatment of concomitant BPH
- Reliable PSA suppression to unrecordable levels
- Decreased patient anxiety during follow-up
- Easy monitoring for recurrent disease
- Radiotherapy possible after surgery

Disadvantages

- Major operation
- Potential mortality (< 0.4%)
- Potential morbidity:
  - impotence (> 50%)
  - persistent incontinence (< 3%)
  - pulmonary embolism (< 1%)
  - rectal injury (< 1%)
  - bladder neck stricture (< 5%)
  - transfusion (20%)

TABLE 4.4 (CONTINUED)

Brachytherapy

Advantages	*Disadvantages*
• One-off treatment	• Cannot be used after previous prostate surgery
• Day-case or overnight procedure	• Limited experience of long-term effects
• Limited period of catheterization	
• Low risk of incontinence	• Difficulty assessing cure
• Lower risk of erectile dysfunction	• Makes subsequent surgery dangerous

seem comparable to open radical prostatectomy. The operating time is usually longer, but blood loss and length of hospital stay is reduced.

Radical prostatectomy, by whichever means achieved, is believed by many urologists to offer the best opportunity for cure in patients with localized prostate cancer. A recent study from Sweden comparing radical prostatectomy with active surveillance confirmed that radical prostatectomy does indeed produce an improvement in prostate-cancer-related mortality; however, the overall survival in the two groups was similar, perhaps because of the age of the patients (64.7 years) and their comorbidity, as well as the relatively short follow-up (6.2 years). As overall survival is the most important parameter, the need for further follow-up is clear. A similar study known as the PIVOT trial is fully recruited in the USA, but results will not be available for some time. Meanwhile, it seems reasonable to discuss the option of radical prostatectomy with younger men with clinically localized disease and no significant comorbidity who have at least a 10-year life expectancy. Thorough counseling as to the potential risks and benefits of radical prostatectomy compared with the other treatment options is essential.

External-beam radiotherapy

External-beam radiotherapy is widely used in the treatment of localized prostate cancer; it offers a particular advantage in patients who are unsuitable candidates for surgery because of either comorbidity or evidence of extraprostatic extension of cancer. Criteria for patients suitable for radiotherapy are shown in Table 4.5. The treatment generally involves a 6-week course of radiotherapy. Survival rates are often comparable to those achieved by radical prostatectomy; several studies have reported 15-year survival rates of 40–60%, even occasionally in patients with relatively advanced disease (stage T3–T4). The principal side effects are urinary frequency and bladder damage, which may occur in a severe form in approximately 2–3% of patients, and rectal irritation producing proctitis and rectal bleeding, which may persist and very occasionally require a colostomy. Erectile dysfunction (ED) due to damage to the neurovascular supply to the corpora cavernosa can also occur, typically over a 6–18 month period. Conformal radiotherapy, which uses new technology to focus the radiation beam more precisely, has recently been introduced; enhanced therapeutic results can be achieved with a lower incidence of side effects. Data from randomized studies continue to suggest that the effect of radiotherapy on locally advanced prostate cancer can be enhanced by 3 months' pretreatment with hormone ablation therapy using an LHRH analog. The advantages and disadvantages of radiotherapy are summarized in Table 4.4 and compared with those of radical prostatectomy and brachytherapy.

Brachytherapy

This technique involves placing either iodine-125 or palladium-103 seeds into the prostate via the transperineal route, using a template and TRUS guidance (Figure 4.2). Brachytherapy carries a low morbidity, and early results confirm satisfactory PSA suppression for 7–10 years at

TABLE 4.5

Selection criteria for radiotherapy in prostate cancer patients

- Histological evidence of prostate cancer
- Regionally localized disease
- Sufficient life expectancy to make cure potentially beneficial
- Absence of lower urinary tract disorders (particularly outflow obstruction)
- Absence of colorectal disease

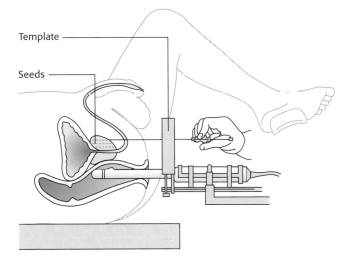

Template ————

Seeds ————

Figure 4.2 Brachytherapy.

least. One recent cohort study, however, has shown a threefold greater risk of recurrence after brachytherapy with palladium-103 in intermediate- and high-risk patients compared with either radical prostatectomy or external beam radiotherapy. Other investigators have reported results equivalent to radical prostatectomy or external-beam radiotherapy. The method is gaining popularity, particularly in the USA. In high-risk patients, brachytherapy may be combined with external-beam radiotherapy to provide a significantly higher radiation dose. The criteria for deciding whether to use both forms of radiotherapy are shown in Table 4.6. Brachytherapy is best avoided in men with severe bladder outflow obstruction because of the swelling of the gland that occurs after seed implantation.

High-intensity focused ultrasound

Recently high-intensity focused ultrasound (HIFU) technology has been developed to treat localized prostate cancer. A specially designed probe delivers HIFU transrectally to the prostate and achieves focal tissue destruction (Figure 4.3). PSA values decline, and responses seem to be maintained. The method should currently be regarded as experimental.

TABLE 4.6

Primary selection criteria for brachytherapy alone versus brachytherapy plus external-beam radiotherapy

	Monotherapy	Combination therapy
Nodule	None or small	Large or multiple
Gleason sum	2–6	7–10
PSA	< 10 ng/mL	≥ 10 ng/mL
Biopsy	Unilateral disease	Bilateral or locally extensive disease
Other criteria	Perineural invasion, age of patient, comorbidities, number or percentage of positive biopsy results, likelihood of understaging or undergrading	

Cryoablation

Freezing temperatures can be used to destroy prostatic tissue. Under TRUS guidance, a number of cryogenic probes are inserted into the prostate via the perineum (Figure 4.4). Liquid nitrogen is then circulated through the probes, producing 'ice balls' with a temperature of approximately –180°C, which disrupt cell membranes, thereby destroying the surrounding tissue. The urethra is protected by circulating warm (44°C) water through a catheter. Although some studies have reported outcomes comparable to those achieved by radical prostatectomy, others have reported an incidence of complications such as rectal and urethral damage. No long-term, randomized, controlled trials have yet compared cryoablation with more established treatments.

Managing recurrence after initial therapy

In spite of treatment either by radical prostatectomy or with radiotherapy (external-beam or brachytherapy), prostate cancer sometimes recurs. The first sign of recurrence is usually a rise in PSA level; this should fall to < 0.1 ng/mL after surgery but usually remains somewhat higher after radiotherapy and other non-invasive treatments.

A sequential rise over a period of months almost always indicates either local or distant recurrence. A high initial PSA value, involved

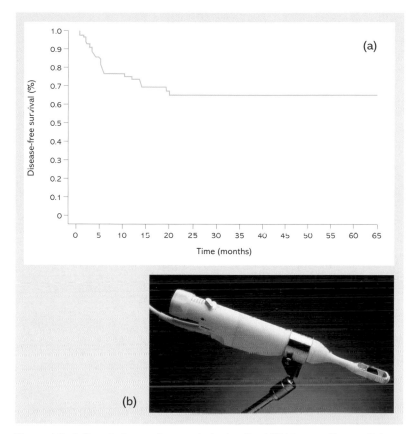

Figure 4.3 a) Overall disease-free survival rate after HIFU therapy. Source: Gelet et al. 2001. b) HIFU probe for endorectal treatment of localized prostate cancer.

seminal vesicles or lymph nodes, positive surgical margins or a Gleason score of > 7 are all risk factors for recurrence.

Staging investigations for suspected recurrence include a transrectal biopsy, which may reveal a residual or recurrent tumor, and a bone scan to detect bone metastases. The Prostascint scan, based on a radioimmunoassay for prostate-specific membrane antigen, may reveal soft tissue metastases, but not infrequently gives false-positive results and is still experimental. A bone scan is usually negative, except in those patients whose recurrence is early and associated with a short PSA doubling time. MRI may reveal the location of soft tissue recurrence.

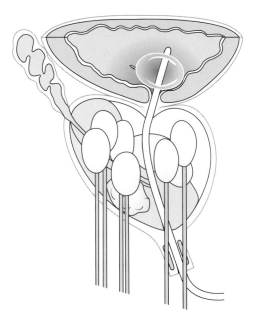

Figure 4.4 In cryoablation, cryogenic probes are inserted into the prostate under ultrasound control, and liquid nitrogen is circulated to destroy prostatic tissue. The urethra is protected by warming through a catheter.

Therapy depends on the original treatment selection. After radical prostatectomy, external-beam radiation may be given, but if the PSA recurrence is rapid and there is a short PSA doubling time, distant metastases are likely and androgen ablation therapy should be considered as an alternative. In cases of recurrence after radiation therapy or brachytherapy, salvage prostatectomy has a high morbidity and is seldom curative; hormonal therapy is usually the better option. Cryotherapy has been advocated by some, and has the advantage of repeatability. Cure in such circumstances is not usually possible, but a prolonged delay in progression is often achieved.

Key points – management of localized disease

- The treatment of localized prostate cancer is controversial.
- Radical prostatectomy probably offers the best long-term prospect of cure, but carries the disadvantage of sexual dysfunction and a mortality of around 0.39%.
- External-beam radiotherapy can be curative, but is associated with an incidence of rectal and bladder complications.
- External beam radiotherapy is more effective when combined with androgen ablation therapy to reduce tumor volume.
- Brachytherapy is gaining in popularity and can be combined with external-beam radiotherapy in high-risk individuals.

Key references

Albertsen PC, Hanley JA, Gleason DF, Barry MJ. Competing risk analysis of men aged 55 to 74 years at diagnosis managed conservatively for clinically localized prostate cancer. *JAMA* 1998;280: 975–80.

Aus G, Pileblad F, Hugosson J. Cryosurgical ablation of the prostate: 5-year follow-up of a prospective study. *Eur Urol* 2002;42:133–8.

Bacon CG, Giovannucci E, Testa M, Kawachi I. The impact of cancer treatment on quality of life outcomes for patients with localized prostate cancer. *J Urol* 2001;166:1804–10.

Blasko JC, Mate T, Sylvester JE et al. Brachytherapy for carcinoma of the prostate: techniques, patient selection, and clinical outcomes. *Semin Radiat Oncol* 2002;12:81–94.

Brawer MK. Treatment of clinically localized prostatic carcinoma: helping our patients make an informed decision [Personal viewpoint]. *Prostate Cancer Prostatic Dis* 2001;4:6–7.

Chodak GW, Thisted RA, Gerber GS et al. Results of conservative management of clinically localized prostate cancer. *N Engl J Med* 1994;4:242–8.

Crook JM, Choan E, Perry GA et al. Serum prostate-specific antigen profile following radiotherapy for prostate cancer: implications for patterns of failure and definition of cure. *Urology* 1998;51:566–72.

D'Amico AV, Whittington R, Malkowicz SB et al. Biochemical outcome after radical prostatectomy, external beam radiation therapy, or interstitial radiation therapy for clinically localized prostate cancer. *JAMA* 1998;280:969–74.

Dearnaley DP, Khoo VS, Norman AR et al. Comparison of radiation side-effects of conformal and conventional radiotherapy and prostate cancer: a randomised trial. *Lancet* 1999;353: 267–72.

Duchesne GM. Radiation for prostate cancer. *Lancet Oncol* 2001;2:73–81.

Epstein JI, Pound CR, Partin AW et al. Disease progression following radical prostatectomy in men with Gleason score 7 tumor. *J Urol* 1998;160:97–101.

Gelet A, Chapelon JY, Bouvier R et al. Transrectal high intensity focused ultrasound for the treatment of localized prostate cancer: factors influencing the outcome. *Eur Urol* 2001;40:124–9.

Graefen M, Karakiewicz PI, Cagiannos I et al. International validation of a preoperative nomogram for prostate cancer recurrence after radical prostatectomy. *J Clin Oncol* 2002;20:3206–12.

Holmberg L, Bill-Axelson A, Helgesen F et al. A randomized trial comparing radical prostatectomy with watchful waiting in early prostate cancer. *N Engl J Med* 2002;347:781–9.

Kirby RS. Treatment options for early prostate cancer. *Urology* 1998;52:948–62.

Klotz LH, Choo R, Morton G, Danjoux C. Expectant management with selective delayed intervention for favorable-risk prostate cancer. *Can J Urol* 2002;9 suppl 1:2–7.

Korb LJ, Brawer MK. Modern brachytherapy for localized prostate cancers: the Northwest Hospital (Seattle) experience. *Rev Urol* 2001;3:51–61.

Langley SE, Laing R. Prostate brachytherapy has come of age: a review of the technique and results. *BJU Int* 2002;89:241–9.

Onik G. Image-guided prostate cryosurgery: state of the art. *Cancer Control* 2001;8:522–31.

Penson DF. Quality of life following prostate cancer treatments. *Curr Urol Rep* 2000;1:71–7.

Pound CR, Partin AW, Eisenberger MA. Natural history of progression after PSA elevation following radical prostatectomy. *JAMA* 1999;281:1591–7.

Ragde H, Elgamal AA, Snow PB et al. Ten-year disease free survival after transperineal sonography-guided iodine-125 brachytherapy with or without 45-gray external-beam irradiation in the treatment of patients with clinically localized, low to high Gleason grade prostate carcinoma. *Cancer* 1998;83: 989–1001.

Salomon L, Levrel O, de la Taille A et al. Radical prostatectomy by the retropubic, perineal and laparoscopic approach: 12 years of experience in one center. *Eur Urol* 2002;42:104–10.

Sharkey J, Cantor A, Solc Z et al. Brachytherapy versus radical prostatectomy in patients with clinically localized prostate cancer. *Curr Urol Rep* 2002;3:250–7.

Sinha AA, Quast BJ, Wilson MJ et al. Prediction of pelvic lymph node metastasis by the ratio of cathepsin B to stefin A in patients with prostate carcinoma. *Cancer* 2002;94:3141–9.

Soffen EM, Hanks GE, Hwang CC et al. Conformal static field therapy for low grade prostate cancer with rigid immobilization. *Int J Radiat Biol Phys* 1992;24:485–8.

Stanford JL, Feng Z, Hamilton AS et al. Urinary and sexual function after radical prostatectomy for clinically localized prostate cancer: the Prostate Cancer Outcomes Study. *JAMA* 2000;283:354–60.

Stone NN, Stock RG. Permanent seed implantation for localized adenocarcinoma of the prostate. *Curr Urol Rep* 2002;3:201–6.

Tewari A, Peabody J, Sarle R et al. Technique of da Vinci robot-assisted anatomic radical prostatectomy. *Urology* 2002;60:569–72.

Walsh PC. Surgery and the reduction of mortality from prostate cancer. *N Engl J Med* 2002;347:839–40.

Wilt TJ. Clarifying uncertainty regarding detection and treatment of early-stage prostate cancer. *Semin Urol Oncol* 2002;20:10–17.

Wilt TJ, Brawer MK. The prostate cancer intervention versus observation trial (PIVOT). *Oncology* 1997;11:1133–43.

Zisman A, Pantuck AJ, Cohen JK, Belldegrun AS. Prostate cryoablation using direct transperineal placement of ultrathin probes through a 17-gauge brachytherapy template-technique and preliminary results. *Urology* 2001;58:988–93.

The term 'locally advanced' prostate cancer classically refers to stage T3N0M0 disease, in which the tumor is no longer confined to the prostate, but there is no clinical evidence of spread to local lymph nodes or more distant sites. However, a more appropriate concern may be prostate cancer with poor prognostic factors, exemplified in Table 5.1. Owing to the imprecision of all local staging techniques, T3N0M0 cancers are often incorrectly staged. The available treatment options are listed in Table 5.2.

Active surveillance

Many patients with locally advanced disease are elderly, and thus have a relatively short life expectancy. Active surveillance may be a valid treatment option in these patients, who will not infrequently succumb to other comorbid conditions. Patients and their immediate family should be fully informed about the implications of opting for deferred therapy, however, and PSA values should be monitored carefully.

Hormonal treatment followed by surgery

Hormonal therapy (cytoreduction) for prostate cancer can normally be achieved by administration of luteinizing-hormone-releasing hormone (LHRH) agonists together with an antiandrogen to prevent initial androgen stimulation of the tumor ('tumor flare'), thereby reducing the

TABLE 5.1

Poor prognostic factors in prostate cancer

- Gleason sum ≥ 8
- Positive seminal vesicle (pT3b)
- Invasion of adjacent structures (pT4)
- Nodal metastases (N1)
- Extensive positive surgical margins

TABLE 5.2

Treatment options for locally advanced prostate cancer

- Active surveillance (watchful waiting)
- Hormonal therapy followed by radiotherapy
- Hormonal therapy followed by surgery
- Hormonal treatment alone
  - LHRH analogs
  - antiandrogen monotherapy
- Intermittent hormonal therapy

tumor burden. This is sometimes referred to as hormonal downstaging. Such treatment has been shown to reduce PSA levels, prostate volume and tumor volume (Figure 5.1). Some studies have demonstrated pathological downstaging after endocrine treatment, but this may be partly attributable to poor initial staging of the tumor or difficulties with pathological interpretation. At present, therefore, androgen ablation therapy as a neoadjuvant prior to radical prostatectomy remains an investigational approach pursued by few clinicians. So far, no survival advantage has been reported for this approach, although the incidence of positive surgical margins does appear to be reduced.

Hormonal therapy followed by radiotherapy

External-beam radiation alone is often inadequate to suppress PSA to within the normal range and prevent disease progression in patients with locally advanced disease. This has led to attempts to use endocrine therapy with an LHRH analog and an antiandrogen as an adjuvant treatment prior to radiotherapy. Reduction of the tumor burden ('downsizing') by endocrine therapy may increase the likelihood of total destruction of the remaining cancer cells by irradiation. This approach is currently being evaluated in randomized trials and increased time to progression has already been reported. In 1997, Bolla et al. reported improved disease-specific survival after continued androgen ablation and radiotherapy compared with radiotherapy alone. Similar results were seen in a North American trial in which recurrence of high PSA

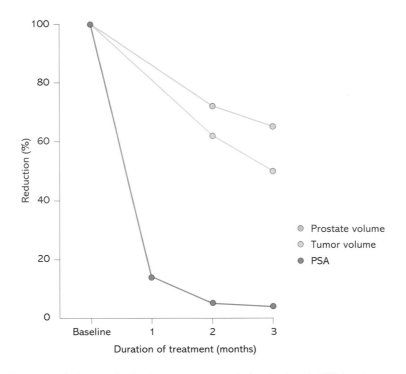

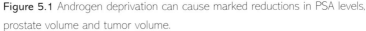

Figure 5.1 Androgen deprivation can cause marked reductions in PSA levels, prostate volume and tumor volume.

levels was seen in 46% of men receiving radiotherapy alone versus 21% of men receiving an LHRH agonist and an antiandrogen in addition to radiation therapy. A recent update on 412 patients with a median follow-up of 66 months by the same author confirmed significant improvements in both disease-free and overall survival in patients receiving LHRH therapy for 3 years after radiotherapy.

Hormonal treatment alone

The development of LHRH analogs and non-steroidal antiandrogens has provided a new generation of endocrine therapies that reduces the intraprostatic concentration of DHT by over 80%. This is comparable to the reduction that can be achieved by surgical orchidectomy. Such treatment reduces tumor volume and delays disease progression in up to 80% of patients with locally advanced prostate cancer. Androgen ablation leads to programmed cell death (apoptosis) in androgen-sensitive cells, but does not completely eliminate malignant cells.

Conventional hormone ablation therapy for locally advanced prostate cancer involves the use of depot LHRH analogs, preceded and accompanied by an antiandrogen for at least 2–6 weeks and sometimes continued thereafter for a variable period of up to 3 years.

Monotherapy with antiandrogens. Recently it has become apparent that monotherapy with the antiandrogen bicalutamide at 150 mg/day can be just as effective in controlling locally advanced disease as castration treatment either by orchidectomy or use of an LHRH analog. A very large international trial has clearly demonstrated delay in objective progression (non-PSA endpoint) in men treated with bicalutamide, 150 mg/day, vs placebo by 42% (Figure 5.2).

The advantage of using the antiandrogen option is that sexual interest and function may be preserved (Figure 5.3). Younger patients may often opt for treatment that has a lesser impact on this important aspect of their lives.

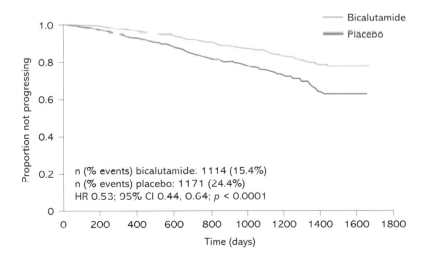

Figure 5.2 Bicalutamide as immediate therapy reduces risk for objective disease progression. Source: See et al. 2002.

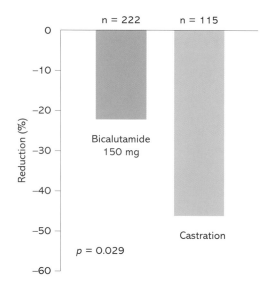

Figure 5.3 Percentage reduction from baseline in sexual interest after 12 months' treatment: bicalutamide, 150 mg, versus castration in M0 patients. Modified with permission from Iversen 1999.

Intermittent hormonal therapy

It has been suggested that continuous androgen ablation therapy may in fact increase the rate of progression of prostate cancer to an androgen-independent state (see Chapter 7). For this reason, attention is currently focused on the use of intermittent hormonal therapy. In this approach, endocrine treatment is given for approximately 36 weeks, provided the PSA is within the normal range at 32 weeks, and then temporarily discontinued. Endocrine treatment is resumed when the serum PSA concentration returns to pretreatment levels in patients with a PSA at diagnosis of < 20 ng/mL, or when PSA increases to > 20 ng/mL in patients with an initial PSA greater than this figure. Such a regimen allows serum testosterone to return to normal, thereby stimulating atrophic cells and rendering them more sensitive to androgen ablation (Figure 5.4). The use of a pure LHRH antagonist, which blocks the receptor without initial stimulation, could be advantageous in this setting owing to the absence of flare and potentially a more rapid restoration of testosterone level after cessation of therapy. In some studies of intermittent hormonal therapy, up to five treatment cycles have been given before evidence of androgen independence has appeared. Randomized trials of intermittent androgen therapy are currently being undertaken and, until these results are available, the approach should be regarded as investigational. However, what appears to be happening is that patients on intermittent therapy are not suffering disease progression any faster than those receiving continuous androgen suppression, and they enjoy improvement in quality of life.

Management of local complications

Locally advanced prostate cancer may precipitate any of several urologic emergencies. Either acute or chronic urinary retention may require TURP. Care should be taken with this procedure not to induce urinary incontinence because the normal landmarks can be distorted by the tumor. A period of catheter drainage while androgen ablation has a chance to relieve the obstruction, followed by a trial without catheter, is often indicated. Anuria due to bilateral ureteric obstruction, either at the vesico-ureteric junction or at the pelvic brim due to enlarged lymph nodes, may necessitate insertion of nephrostomy tubes or passage of a double-pigtail stent and subsequent external-beam radiotherapy. Bleeding from the tumor may occasionally precipitate hematuria and

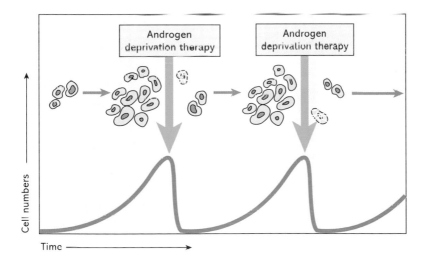

Figure 5.4 Intermittent androgen ablation therapy allows serum testosterone to return periodically to normal, thereby stimulating atrophic cells and rendering them sensitive to subsequent androgen ablation.

clot retention requiring bladder washout and irrigation, and sometimes diathermy or even embolization of bleeding tumor vessels.

Key points – management of locally advanced disease

- Locally advanced prostate cancer is characterized by local tumor spread beyond the prostate without distant metastases.
- Local staging by MRI may be helpful but is subject to inaccuracies.
- Treatment with a combination of hormonal downsizing followed by external-beam radiotherapy is more effective than radiotherapy alone.
- A recent large international trial confirmed that treatment with the antiandrogen bicalutamide, 150 mg/day, reduced objective progression by 42%.

Key references

Bolla M, Collette L, Blank L et al. Long-term results with immediate androgen suppression and external irradiation in patients with locally advanced prostate cancer (an EORTC study): a phase III randomised trial. *Lancet* 2002;360:103–6.

Bolla M, Gonzalez D, Warde P et al. Improved survival in patients with locally advanced prostate cancer treated with radiotherapy and goserelin. *N Engl J Med* 1997; 337:295–300.

Brawer MK. The evolution of hormonal therapy for prostatic carcinoma. *Rev Urol* 2001; 3(suppl 3):S1–S9.

Brawer MK. Bicalutamide as immediate therapy either alone or as adjuvant to the standard care of patients with localized or locally advanced prostate cancer: first analysis of the Early Prostate Cancer program. *BJU Int* 2003;91:465–6.

Chawla AK, Thakral HK, Zietman AL, Shipley WU. Salvage radiotherapy after radical prostatectomy for prostate adenocarcinoma: analysis of efficacy and prognostic factors. *Urology* 2002;59:726–31.

Gleave ME, Goldenberg L, Jones EC. Biochemical and pathological effects of 8 months of neoadjuvant androgen withdrawal therapy before radical prostatectomy in patients with clinically confined prostate cancer. *J Urol* 1996;155:213–19.

Goldenberg SL, Bruchovsky N, Gleave ME et al. Intermittent androgen suppression in the treatment of prostate cancer: a preliminary report. *Urology* 1994;45:839–45.

Hellerstedt BA, Pienta KJ. The current state of hormonal therapy for prostate cancer. *CA Cancer J Clin* 2002;52:154–79.

Iversen P. Quality of life issues relating to endocrine treatment options. *Eur Urol* 1999;36 (suppl 2):20–6.

Iversen P. Antiandrogen monotherapy: indications and results. *Urology* 2002;60(3 suppl 1):64–71.

Klein EA, Kupelian PA, Dreicer R et al. Locally advanced prostate cancer. *Curr Treat Options Oncol* 2001;2:403–11.

Mayer R, Pummer K, Quehenberger F et al. Postprostatectomy radiotherapy for high-risk prostate cancer. *Urology* 2002;59:732–9.

Pilepich MV, Sause WF, Shipley WU et al. Androgen deprivation with radiation therapy compared with radiation therapy alone for locally advanced prostatic carcinoma: a randomized comparative trial of the Radiation Therapy Oncology Group. *Urology* 1995;45:616–23.

Pound CW, Brawer MK, Partin AW. Evaluation and treatment of men with biochemical prostate specific antigen recurrence following definitive therapy for clinically localized prostate cancer. *Rev Urol* 2001;3:72–84.

See WA, Wirth MP, McLeod DG et al. Bicalutamide as immediate therapy either alone or as adjuvant to standard care of patients with localized or locally advanced prostate cancer: first analysis of the early prostate cancer program. *J Urol* 2002;168.429–35.

Wirth M, Tyrrell C, Wallace M et al. Bicalutamide (Casodex) 150 mg as immediate therapy in patients with localized or locally advanced prostate cancer significantly reduces the risk of disease progression. *Urology* 2001; 58:146–51.

Although there is an increasing tendency towards early detection of prostate cancer, many patients throughout the world still present with metastatic disease. In countries where PSA testing is not widely utilized, around 30% of patients currently present with localized disease, 40% with locally advanced disease and the remaining 30% with metastases. In contrast to localized or locally advanced disease, metastatic prostate cancer is associated with high mortality – approximately 70% within 5 years. Androgen deprivation, either by orchidectomy or treatment with LHRH analogs, remains the mainstay of treatment (Table 6.1), though the value of maximal androgen blockade (LHRH agonist + antiandrogen) is still debated. Pure LHRH antagonists are currently under investigation, but are not yet approved by regulatory authorities.

Orchidectomy

Bilateral orchidectomy or bilateral subcapsular orchidectomy is performed through a midline scrotal incision (Figure 6.1) under local, regional or light general anesthetic. The procedure is simple and is associated with little morbidity. The principal adverse events that may occur after orchidectomy are local complications such as hematoma and wound infections, together with loss of libido, ED and hot flashes. Clinical responses (decreased bone pain and reduced PSA concentration) are obtained in more than 75% of patients. Because of

TABLE 6.1

Treatment options for metastatic prostate cancer

- Androgen deprivation
  - orchidectomy
  - LHRH analogs
- Maximal androgen blockade

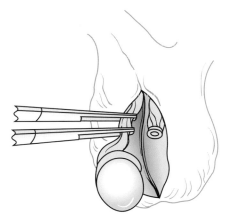

Figure 6.1 Bilateral orchidectomy is generally performed via a midline scrotal incision.

the psychological and cosmetic impact of orchidectomy, however, most patients prefer reversible non-surgical treatment with LHRH analogs.

LHRH analogs

LHRH analogs, such as goserelin acetate, buserelin and leuprolide, are highly potent LHRH agonists (superagonists). After administration, there is a transient initial increase in LH secretion, and hence in testosterone secretion; this is followed by desensitization (downregulation), resulting in a fall in LH and testosterone secretion (Figure 6.2). These agents are usually given as 1- or 3-monthly depot preparations, which are administered subcutaneously in the abdominal area. A potential side effect is the tumor 'flare' that 8–32% of patients experience as a result of the initial transient increase (140–170%) in testosterone. This may result in increased bone pain or worsening of symptoms of bladder outflow obstruction; spinal metastases may also be stimulated, producing a risk of spinal cord compression. Tumor flare can be avoided by prior and concomitant administration of an antiandrogen during the first 6 weeks of treatment. Comparative trials have shown that the response rates obtained with LHRH analogs are equivalent to those obtained after orchidectomy, in terms of both time to progression and overall survival.

LHRH antagonists

Recently, pure LHRH antagonists have been developed and tested. These peptides inhibit LHRH release without initial stimulation by blocking pituitary receptors and thus are not associated with a surge in testosterone (flare). This results in more rapid achievement of the castrate state. More rapid return of testosterone with intermittent application is potentially an additional benefit. However, none of these agents are currently licensed for clinical use.

Maximal androgen blockade

Although both orchidectomy and LHRH treatment produce dramatic initial responses in 70–80% of patients, remission is not usually maintained in the long term. Androgen-independent cancer cell clones are selected out, so the mean time to tumor progression is less than

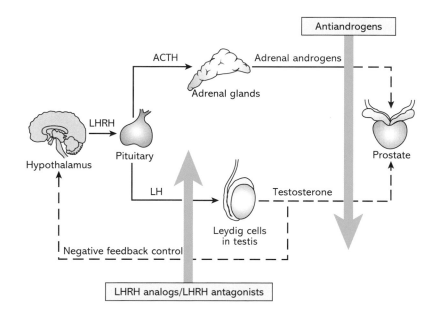

Figure 6.2 LHRH analogs inhibit pituitary LH secretion, and thus reduce testicular androgen secretion. Antiandrogens act peripherally to block testosterone action on androgen receptors. ACTH, adrenocorticotropic hormone.

18 months and the mean overall survival time is approximately 28–36 months. One factor that may contribute to this poor prognosis is persistent adrenal androgen secretion; there is evidence that adrenal androgens account for up to 15–20% of total androgen concentrations within the prostate. This has led to the concept of maximal androgen blockade, in which androgen deprivation by orchidectomy or LHRH treatment is accompanied by treatment with an antiandrogen to block the effects of adrenal androgens in the prostate.

Maximal androgen blockade with a combination of a LHRH analog and an antiandrogen has been shown in several trials to offer improved survival compared with either LHRH treatment alone (Figure 6.3) or orchidectomy (Figure 6.4). Other trials, however, have failed to show

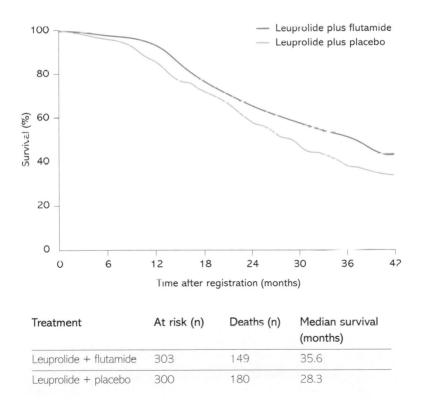

Treatment	At risk (n)	Deaths (n)	Median survival (months)
Leuprolide + flutamide	303	149	35.6
Leuprolide + placebo	300	180	28.3

Figure 6.3 Maximal androgen blockade has been reported to improve survival compared with LHRH treatment alone. Data from Crawford ED et al. 1989.

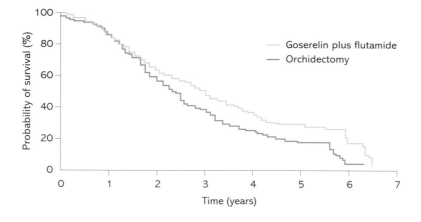

Figure 6.4 Maximal androgen blockade with an LHRH analog and an antiandrogen has been reported to lead to improved survival compared with orchidectomy. Data from Denis et al. 1993.

significant improvements in tumor progression and survival, and a meta-analysis of all studies failed to confirm definitively an advantage of combined therapy. The reasons for this discrepancy may include short follow-up times and the presence of tumor flare effects in patients treated with LHRH analogs without concomitant initial antiandrogen therapy. At present, it appears that maximal androgen blockade may offer a slight advantage over monotherapy, at least in a subgroup of patients with good performance status (i.e. those who are generally well in themselves) and a relatively restricted metastatic burden. Such treatment should therefore be considered in younger and fitter patients who are most likely to die from prostate cancer itself rather than from some comorbid condition. However, the relatively modest benefits do need to be weighed against the costs and small but significant incidence of side effects from the antiandrogen.

The timing of initiating hormonal therapy has been the subject of vigorous debate; recently the evidence seems to favor earlier therapy rather than waiting for symptoms. This evidence includes a reanalysis of the VA cooperative studies (USA) in which men receiving 1 mg of diethylstilbestrol had a survival advantage. The Medical Research

Council (UK) study showed men with locally advanced or metastatic disease treated with castration at the time of diagnosis had better outcomes than those receiving deferred therapy (Figure 6.5), and a US trial reported by Messing et al. found that men with pelvic lymph-node metastases treated with delayed hormonal therapy had a sevenfold greater rate of prostate cancer death than those who had immediate androgen ablation therapy.

Spinal cord compression and pathological fractures

Sudden onset of low back pain and weakness in the lower limbs, with or without voiding difficulty, in a patient with metastatic prostate cancer should be considered to be a urologic/neurosurgical emergency. Spinal cord compression, due to pathological fracture or collapse of the lumbar vertebrae, is the most common reason for these symptoms (Figure 6.6). The diagnosis may be confirmed by urgent spinal MRI. Early neurosurgical decompression is often advised, usually followed by external-beam radiotherapy and corticosteroids.

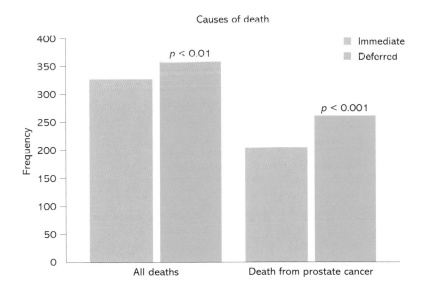

Figure 6.5 Immediate versus deferred treatment for advanced prostate cancer (Data: Medical Research Council 1997).

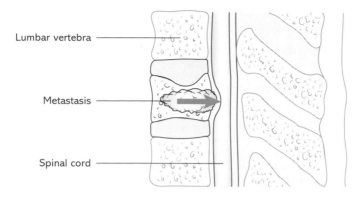

Lumbar vertebra

Metastasis

Spinal cord

Figure 6.6 Spinal cord compression as a result of a spinal metastasis.

Pathological fractures due to prostate cancer metastases may occur elsewhere, for example in the femur or humerus. Fixation by an orthopedic specialist is often required and should usually be followed by external-beam radiotherapy and androgen ablation.

Key points – management of metastatic disease

- Metastatic prostate cancer is characterized by a positive bone scan and/or the presence of soft-tissue metastases.
- PSA values are usually high, often > 50 ng/mL.
- Treatment is usually by androgen ablation.
- An LHRH analog preceded and then accompanied by an antiandrogen is the most frequently employed treatment strategy.
- Responses in terms of PSA reduction and clinical improvement are seen in > 80% of patients.
- Eventually, however, androgen-insensitive cell clones develop and the PSA level begins to rise.

Key references

Crawford ED, Eisenberger MA, McLeod DG et al. A controlled trial of leuprolide with and without flutamide in prostatic carcinoma. *N Engl J Med* 1989;321: 419–24.

Denis LD, Carneiro de Moura JL, Bono A et al. Goserelin acetate and flutamide versus bilateral orchidectomy: a phase III EORTC trial (30853). *Urology* 1993;42:119–29.

Errejon A, Crawford ED. Monotherapy versus combined androgen blockade in patients with advanced prostate cancer. *Cancer* 2002;95:209–10.

Iversen P. Quality of life issues relating to endocrine treatment options. *Eur Urol* 1999;36 (suppl 2):20 6.

Janknegt RA, Abbou CC, Bartoletti R et al. Orchidectomy and nilutamide or placebo as treatment of metastatic prostatic cancer in a multinational double-blind randomised trial. *J Urol* 1993;149:77–83.

Medical Research Council Prostate Cancer Working Party Investigators Group. Immediate versus deferred treatment for advanced prostate cancer: initial results of the MRC Trial. *Br J Urol* 1997;79:235–46.

Messing EM, Manola J, Sarosdy M et al. Immediate hormonal therapy compared with observation after radical prostatectomy and pelvic lymphadenopathy in men with node-positive prostate cancer. *N Engl J Med* 1999;341:1781–8.

Mittan D, Lee S, Miller E et al. Bone loss following hypogonadism in men with prostate cancer treated with GnRH analogs. *J Clin Endocrinol Metab* 2002;87:3656–61.

Prostate Cancer Trialists Collaborative Group. Maximum androgen blockade in advanced prostate cancer: an overview of 22 randomized trials with 3283 deaths in 5710 patients. *Lancet* 1995;346:265–9.

Schellhammer PF, Sharifi R, Block NL et al. A controlled trial of bicalutamide versus flutamide, each in combination with luteinizing hormone-releasing hormone analog therapy in patients with advanced prostate cancer. *Urology* 1995; 45:745–51.

Schellhammer PF, Sharifi R, Block NL. Clinical benefits of bicalutamide compared with flutamide in combined androgen blockade for patients with advanced prostatic carcinoma: final report of a double-blind, randomized multicentre trial. *Urology* 1997;50:330–6.

Tyrrell CJ, Denis L, Newling D et al. Casodex™ 10–200 mg daily used as monotherapy for the treatment of patients with advanced prostate cancer. An overview of the efficacy, tolerability and pharmacokinetics from three phase II dose-ranging studies. Casodex Study Group. *Eur Urol* 1998;33:39–53.

Management of androgen-independent disease

In almost all cases, advanced prostate cancers treated with any form of androgen ablation eventually begin to progress, a phenomenon known as 'hormone escape' or androgen independence. This is probably due either to clonal selection of androgen-independent cell lines (Figure 7.1) or to increased ligand-independent activation of androgen receptors. Thus, an increase in PSA level after initially successful androgen ablation almost inevitably indicates impending clinical progression. Until recently, therapy had little impact beyond modest palliation; however, a number of second-line treatments that may delay the progression of symptoms and reduce serum PSA are becoming available (Table 7.1).

Antiandrogen withdrawal

When the serum PSA level rises after a period of androgen ablation therapy, an initial move that may be beneficial in some patients is

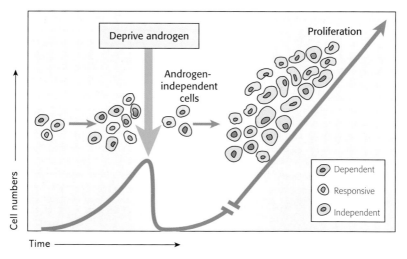

Figure 7.1 Hormone escape results from the selection of androgen-independent cell lines.

TABLE 7.1

Second-line treatments for androgen-independent prostate cancer

- Antiandrogen withdrawal
- Cytotoxic chemotherapy
- Hormonal or chemohormonal therapy
- Combination cytotoxic and chemohormonal therapy
- Experimental approaches:
  - growth factor signal inhibition
  - antisense oligonucleotides
  - monoclonal antibodies and targeted gene vectors

withdrawal of the antiandrogen treatment. A favorable PSA response is sometimes seen. This phenomenon (which also occurs in breast cancer treated with antiestrogens) has been ascribed to a mutation of androgen receptors in malignant tissue that renders the antiandrogen an agonist rather than an antagonist in effect.

Cytotoxic therapy

Cytotoxic therapy in prostate cancer produces good PSA responses and delays time to progression, but proven overall survival benefit remains elusive. Mitoxantrone plus hydrocortisone, for example, increased time to progression in a study of 242 patients (Kantoff et al.), but overall survival was around 12 months in both groups.

So far docetaxel (Taxotere) is the most promising single cytotoxic agent, dosed either weekly or 3-weekly. Table 7.2 summarizes the evidence for the efficacy of docetaxel. Side effects include neutropenia, skin reactions and gastrointestinal problems, but in general the drug is well tolerated.

Estrogens

Estrogen treatment may be beneficial in some patients with androgen-independent prostate cancer. Such treatment appears to have two effects:

- inhibition of pituitary gonadotropin secretion
- direct cytotoxic effect on the tumor.

TABLE 7.2

Clinical trials with single-agent docetaxel in hormone-refractory prostate cancer

Study	Docetaxel regimen	Number of evaluable patients	PSA decline > 50%	Measurable disease response
Picus 1999	75 mg/m² every 3 weeks	35	46%	28% (7/25)
Friedland 1999	75 mg/m² every 3 weeks	16	38%	60% (6/10)
Berry 2001	36 mg/m²/week × 6 of an 8-week cycle	59	41%	33% (2/6)
Beer 2001	36 mg/m²/week × 6 of an 8-week cycle	24	46%	40% (2/5)

The synthetic estrogen diethylstilbestrol (DES) has been used in prostate cancer, but its use as first-line therapy is limited by side effects such as gynecomastia, deep-vein thrombosis and other cardiovascular complications. Combination of DES with aspirin may reduce thrombotic and cardiovascular toxicity that can be hazardous in men of this age.

Estramustine phosphate combines a nitrogen mustard with phosphorylated estradiol and is currently attracting some attention as a second-line treatment for prostate cancer. It is metabolized to estrogenic compounds, but its primary cytotoxic action is disruption of microtubules, resulting in blockade of cell division and ultimately cell death. Phase II trials have produced objective response rates of 30–35%. Smith et al. reported that estramustine had similar efficacy to DES, with less cardiovascular but more gastrointestinal toxicity.

Cytotoxic/chemohormonal combination therapy

Currently this treatment appears to hold the greatest promise for patients with androgen-independent prostate cancer. Table 7.3 summarizes the results of the phase II studies reported to date. Two large, randomized phase III studies, one of docetaxel and estramustine,

TABLE 7.3

Phase II clinical trials with cytotoxic/chemohormonal combination therapy in hormone-refractory prostate cancer

Study	Agents used	Number of evaluable patients	PSA decline > 50%
Beer 2003	Docetaxel + calcitriol	36	81%
Figg 2001	Docetaxel + thalidomide	59	53%
Sweeney 2002	Vinorelbine + estramustine	23	71%
Ellerhorst 1997	Doxorubicin + ketoconazole alternating with vinblastine + estramustine	46	67%

the other of docetaxel and prednisolone, have now completed accrual; results are expected soon.

Inhibition of growth factor signaling and microtubules

A number of growth factors have been shown to be involved in the development and progression of prostate cancer, including:

- epidermal growth factor (EGF)
- insulin like growth factor (IGF)
- platelet-derived growth factor (PDGF)
- fibroblast growth factor (FGF).

Recognition of the importance of growth factors in prostate cancer has led to attempts to use growth factor inhibitors in the management of advanced disease. The most widely studied agent is suramin, which blocks the binding of EGF and IGF to their receptors. In preliminary trials, this agent has produced promising results, but a wide range of adverse effects, such as skin disorders and neuromuscular toxicity, has been reported.

Most growth factors act via a common intracellular pathway that involves tyrosine kinase. Compounds that inhibit tyrosine kinase might be anticipated to be effective in the treatment of prostate cancer, and one, ZD1839 (Iressa), is currently undergoing investigation in this and other cancers.

Other potential avenues for the future include the use of angiogenesis inhibitors, including thalidomide and angiostatin, which hold considerable promise but are not yet approved by regulatory authorities. Antagonists of endothelin-A, such as atrasentan, appear to have some useful activity, as recently reported by Carducci et al.

Management of bone metastases

Bone pain is one of the most intractable problems associated with androgen-independent prostate cancer, and conventional analgesics may not always provide relief. There is now evidence that some patients may benefit symptomatically from treatment with bisphosphonates, which suppress bone resorption and demineralization. A study involving over 600 patients with hormone-refractory prostate cancer compared

---

Key points – management of androgen-independent disease

- After an initial response to androgen ablation the serum PSA value starts to rise as a result of androgen-insensitive cell clones.
- As an initial maneuver any antiandrogen that the patient is taking should be withdrawn.
- Introduction of low-dose estrogen (such as stilbestrol, 1–3 mg/day) + aspirin may result in a PSA response, but carries a risk of cardiovascular complications.
- Treatment with chemotherapeutic agents has historically been disappointing, but recent studies with mitoxantrone, estramustine and docetaxel look more promising.
- The bisphosphonate zoledronic acid has been reported to delay significantly the occurrence of skeletal events in patients with metastatic prostate cancer.
- A large number of new approaches, including growth-factor signal inhibition and angiogenesis inhibition, are under investigation.

zoledronic acid, given as an intravenous infusion over 15 minutes every 3 weeks, with placebo. There was a significant reduction in the number of patients with skeletal-related events, and the first such event was significantly delayed (Figure 7.2), in the bisphosphonate-treated arm. External-beam radiotherapy may also be useful, bringing effective localized pain relief to 70–80% of patients when given either as a single dose or in short (2–3 week) courses. Wide-field radiation may also be useful in patients with intractable diffuse pain, but this approach produces nausea, vomiting and diarrhea in approximately 35% of patients, and severe, sometimes irreversible, hematological effects in 9%. Intravenous administration of radioactive isotopes that have a high affinity for the skeleton, such as strontium-89, constitutes a valuable advance in the palliation of metastatic disease. Strontium-89 is given by single intravenous injection, and may significantly reduce the need for other analgesic agents for as long as 6 months. The major side effects are neutropenia and granulocytopenia; white blood cell count and platelet levels should be monitored before and after therapy.

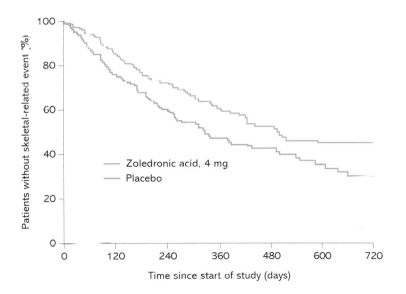

Figure 7.2 Kaplan–Meier estimates of event rates for time to the first skeletal-related event for patients with metastatic prostate cancer randomized to receive zoledronic acid or placebo. Data: Saad et al. 2003.

Despite improving second-line therapy, most patients with metastatic prostate cancer will eventually die as a result of the disease, often in 12–24 months of developing androgen independence. Treatment with high-dose steroids can sometimes provide useful palliation. The palliative care of these patients requires a supportive and caring team approach, involving the family physician, the urologist, an experienced palliative care team and, of course, the patient's close relatives.

Key references

Beer TM, Eilers KM, Garzotto M et al. Weekly high-dose calcitriol and docetaxel in metastatic androgen-independent prostate cancer. *J Clin Oncol* 2003;21:123–8.

Beer TM, Pierce WC, Lowe BA, Henner WD. Phase II study of weekly docetaxel in symptomatic androgen-independent prostate cancer. *Ann Oncol* 2001;12:1273–9.

Berry W, Dakhil S, Gregurich MA, Asmar L. Phase II trial of single-agent weekly docetaxel in hormone-refractory, symptomatic, metastatic carcinoma of the prostate. *Semin Oncol* 2001;28(4 suppl 15):8–15.

Carducci MA, Padley RJ, Breul J et al. Effect of endothelin-A receptor blockade with atrasentan on tumor progression in men with hormone-refractory prostate cancer: a randomized, phase II, placebo-controlled trial. *J Clin Oncol* 2003; 21:679–89.

Ellerhorst JA, Tu SM, Amato RJ et al. Phase II trial of alternating weekly chemohormonal therapy for patients with androgen-independent prostate cancer. *Clin Cancer Res* 1997;3: 2371–6.

Figg WD, Arlen P, Gulley J et al. A randomized phase II trial of docetaxel (Taxotere) plus thalidomide in androgen-independent prostate cancer. *Semin Oncol* 2001; 28(4 suppl 15):62–6.

Friedland D, Cohen J, Miller R Jr et al. A phase II trial of docetaxel (Taxotere) in hormone-refractory prostate cancer: correlation of antitumor effect to phosphorylation of Bcl-2. *Semin Oncol* 1999; 26(5 suppl 17):19–23.

Gilligan T, Kantoff PW. Chemotherapy for prostate cancer. *Urology* 2002;60(3 suppl 1):94–100.

Hansenson M, Lundh B, Hartley-Asp B, Pousette Å. Growth-inhibiting effect of estramustine on two prostatic carcinoma cell lines, LNCaP and LNCaP-r. *Urol Res* 1988;16:357–61.

Harris KA, Reese DM. Treatment options in hormone-refractory prostate cancer: current and future approaches. *Drugs* 2001;61:2177–92.

Kantoff PW, Halabi S, Conaway M et al. Hydrocortisone with or without mitoxantrone in men with hormone-refractory prostate cancer: results of the cancer and leukemia group B 9182 study. *J Clin Oncol* 1999; 17:2506–13.

Kish JA, Bukkapatnam R, Palazzo F. The treatment challenge of hormone-refractory prostate cancer. *Cancer Control* 2001;8:487–95.

Lewington V, McEwan AJ, Ackery DM et al. A prospective, randomized double-blind crossover study to examine the efficacy of strontium-89 in pain palliation in patients with advanced prostate cancer metastatic to bone. *Eur J Cancer* 1991,27:954–8.

Logothetis CJ. Docetaxel in the integrated management of prostate cancer. Current applications and future promise. *Oncology* 2002; 16(6 suppl 6):63–72.

Marks LS, DiPaola RS, Nelson P et al. PC-SPES: herbal formulation for prostate cancer. *Urology* 2002;60: 369–75; discussion 376–7.

Picus J, Schultz M. Docetaxel (Taxotere) as monotherapy in the treatment of hormone-refractory prostate cancer: preliminary results. *Semin Oncol* 1999; 26(5 suppl 17):14–8.

Saad F, Gleason DM, Murray R et al. Zoledronic acid is well tolerated for up to 24 months and significantly reduces skeletal complications in patients with advanced prostate cancer metastatic to bone. Presented to American Urological Association, 26 April – 1 May 2003. *Proc Am Urol Assoc* 2003;abstract 1472.

Saad F, Gleason DM, Murray R et al. A randomized, placebo-controlled trial of zoledronic acid in patients with hormone-refractory metastatic prostate carcinoma. *J Natl Cancer Inst* 2002;94:1458–68.

Savarese DM, Halabi S, Hars V et al. Phase II study of docetaxel, estramustine, and low-dose hydrocortisone in men with hormone-refractory prostate cancer. A final report of Cancer and Leukemia Group B 9780. *J Clin Oncol* 2001;19:2509–16.

Smith PH, Suciu S, Robinson MR et al. A comparison of the effect of diethylstilbestrol with estramustine phosphate in the treatment of advanced prostatic cancer: final analysis of a phase III trial of the European Organization for Research on Treatment of Cancer. *J Urol* 1986; 136:619–23.

Sweeney CJ, Monaco FJ, Jung SH et al. A phase II Hoosier Oncology Group study of vinorelbine and estramustine phosphate in hormone-refractory prostate cancer. *Ann Oncol* 2002;13:435–40.

The prostate is an androgen-dependent organ which is intimately involved in several aspects of sexual function. Not surprisingly, therefore, prostate cancer itself, and the treatments required either to eradicate it or to delay its progression, often result in sexual dysfunction. The problems encountered, which may be isolated or combined, can be categorized as:

- ED
- ejaculatory and orgasmic disturbance
- loss of libido.

A diagnosis of prostate cancer alone may be enough to disturb sex lives that, in the age group usually affected, are often already waning. In one survey, a surprising number of couples erroneously believed that prostate cancer could be sexually transmitted; they therefore voluntarily abstained from sex. This highlights the need for all those involved in the care of prostate cancer patients to discuss sexual function openly, not only with the sufferer, but also with his partner. It is often helpful to provide patients with written information to take home and study, and an opportunity for them to return to deal with any queries that arise.

The effect of treatment

Almost all treatments aimed at eradicating localized prostate cancer carry a risk of inducing ED; tumescence is the most vulnerable aspect of male sexual function. Radical retropubic prostatectomy is most often implicated in this respect. The nerve-sparing modification described by Walsh, as well as intraoperative nerve stimulation and sural nerve grafting, have significantly reduced the incidence of ED.

External-beam radiotherapy and brachytherapy are both associated with an incidence of ED of 30% or more. Cryotherapy very often results in ED because the neurovascular bundles are included in the freezing zone. Loss of ejaculation may also occur after transurethral surgery for local disease. Loss of libido is very common with androgen ablation therapy for more advanced disease.

Erectile dysfunction

Erectile dysfunction resulting from prostate cancer therapy can be treated safely and reasonably effectively in most cases. There is now evidence that early institution of treatment may help prevent the development of intracorporeal fibrosis, which results from the release of transforming growth factor-α (TGF-α). As TGF-α is released in response to anoxia, therapies that bring oxygenated arterial blood into the corpora and induce erection inhibit its release and may help maintain smooth muscle function.

Treatment options include the use of vacuum devices, though some couples find them cumbersome and lacking in spontaneity. New oral therapies, such as the phosphodiesterase type 5 inhibitors sildenafil, tadalafil and vardenafil (the latter two more recently developed and now licensed in most countries), and intraurethral or intracavernosal prostaglandin E1 are often more acceptable. Sublingual apomorphine, 3 mg, may sometimes help. α-blockers, such as doxazosin or alfuzosin taken orally, can also be mildly beneficial, possibly acting by reducing the sympathetic vasoconstriction of the intracavernosal vasculature, and may work in conjunction with the vasodilatory action of a phosphodiesterase type 5 inhibitor or prostaglandin E1. As yet, they are not licensed for this indication.

Ejaculatory disturbance

Ejaculatory disorders may occur in prostate cancer as a result of prostatic surgery. Both TURP, performed for outflow obstruction caused by the tumor, and radical prostatectomy are associated with ejaculatory disturbance, though sensation of orgasm is usually preserved. In the case of TURP, semen is still produced, but passes retrogradely into the bladder. After radical prostatectomy, in which the entire prostate and seminal vesicles have been removed, no semen is produced, but most patients are still able to achieve orgasm. Patients must be informed about these consequences before surgery. Drugs such as the $\alpha1$-blocker tamsulosin, used to treat bladder outflow obstruction, may also cause retrograde ejaculation, but this is reversible on cessation of treatment.

> **Key points – sexual function and prostate cancer**
>
> - Sexual dysfunction is a common sequela to prostate cancer treatment.
> - The implications should be discussed with the patient and his partner.
> - Erectile dysfunction can often be improved with phosphodiesterase type 5 inhibitors, prostaglandin suppositories or injections, or mechanical vacuum devices.
> - Loss of libido can be reduced by using antiandrogens as opposed to bilateral orchidectomy or an LHRH analog to treat prostate cancer.

Loss of libido

Loss of libido is a common complaint of patients with prostate cancer. It may result from the disease itself causing debilitation or depression. More commonly, it is a side effect of hormone ablation therapy. Bilateral orchidectomy or therapy with LHRH analogs is almost invariably associated with loss of libido, as well as ED. Therapy with an antiandrogen can effectively deprive prostate cancer cells of androgen stimulation without such a profound effect on libido or erectile function.

If preservation of sexual function is an important factor in terms of the quality of life of an individual prostate cancer sufferer, then treatment with an antiandrogen as monotherapy may well be considered as an alternative to bilateral orchidectomy or an LHRH analog.

Counseling

The most important conclusion to be drawn is that patients with prostate cancer, as well as their partners, should be counseled not only about probable outcomes, but also about the likely effect of the disease and its therapy on their sex lives. A more open and informed approach to this important aspect of prostate cancer would do much not only to counter the anxiety and loss of self-esteem that so often accompanies the diagnosis of this frequently encountered malignancy, but also restore effective sexual function after treatment.

Key references

Carson CC, Burnett AL, Levine LA, Nehra A. The efficacy of sildenafil citrate (Viagra) in clinical populations: an update. *Urology* 2002;60(2 suppl 2):12–27.

Fitzpatrick JM, Kirby RS, Krane RJ et al. Sexual dysfunction associated with the management of prostate cancer. *Eur Urol* 1998;33:513–22.

Goldstein I, Lue TF, Padma-Nathan H. Oral sildenafil in the treatment of erectile dysfunction. *N Engl J Med* 1998;338:1397–404.

Heaton JP. Characterising the benefit of apomorphine SL (Uprima) as an optimised treatment for representative populations with erectile dysfunction *Int J Impot Res* 2001;13 suppl 3:S35–9.

Kirby RS, Watson A, Newling DWW. Prostate cancer and sexual function. *Prostate Cancer Prostatic Diseases* 1998;1:179–84.

Padma-Nathan H, Hellstrom WJ, Kaiser FF et al. Treatment of men with erectile dysfunction with transurethral alprostadil Medicated Urethral System for Erection (MUSE). *N Engl J Med* 1997;336:1–7.

Padma-Nathan H, McMurray JG, Pullman WE et al. On-demand IC351 (Cialis) enhances erectile function in patients with erectile dysfunction. *Int J Impot Res* 2001;13:2–9.

Paige NM, Hays RD, Litwin MS et al. Improvement in emotional well-being and relationships of users of sildenafil. *J Urol* 2001;166:1774–8.

Walsh PC, Lepor H, Eggleston JC. Radical prostatectomy with preservation of sexual function: anatomical and pathological considerations, *Prostate* 1983;4: 473–85.

Willke RJ, Glick HA, McCarron TJ et al. Quality of life effects of alprostadil therapy for erectile dysfunction. *J Urol* 1997;157: 2124–8.

Zelefsky MJ, McKee AB, Lee H, Leibel SA. Efficacy of oral sildenafil in patients with erectile dysfunction after radiotherapy for carcinoma of the prostate. *Urology* 1999;53:775–8.

Zippe CD, Jhaveri FM, Klein EA et al. Role of Viagra after radical prostatectomy. *Urology* 2000;55: 241–5.

Until recently, prostate cancer has been something of a Cinderella subject as far as basic research is concerned. Other common neoplasms, such as breast or colorectal cancers, have attracted far greater academic attention and considerably more research funding. Perhaps because of increased public awareness of the potentially devastating effects of prostatic malignancy, this balance is now being redressed. It seems probable that increasing awareness and redoubled research endeavors into prostate cancer will eventually translate into improved survival prospects for the many sufferers of this very prevalent disease.

Chemoprevention

Potentially, prostate cancer should be a preventable disease (Figure 9.1). Already there is some evidence that both vitamin E and selenium may

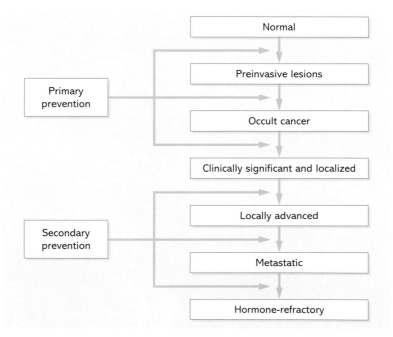

Figure 9.1 Possible prophylactic interventions in prostate cancer.

have some chemopreventative effect. The type II 5α-reductase inhibitor finasteride has also been evaluated in a 7-year randomized trial in 18 882 men. Published results confirm a 24.8% reduction in prostate cancer risk in the group treated with finasteride (Figure 9.2) as well as a reduced incidence of urinary symptoms, although at the cost of a small risk of sexual side effects and a slightly greater incidence of high-grade prostate cancer. However, Gleason grading of prostate cancer has not been validated for use in patients treated with hormonal therapy, because the treatment creates a bias towards higher grades, and consequently may not correlate with tumor aggressiveness in this situation. Several other agents appear promising, but long-term, controlled studies are required to confirm their efficacy in this respect; one, the REDUCE study of the use of the dual 5α-reductase inhibitor dutasteride for chemoprevention, is already under way.

Earlier detection

Earlier detection, when the disease is still curable, is already a reality as a result of PSA testing, and newer assays that can distinguish free from complexed PSA further improve the diagnostic sensitivity and specificity

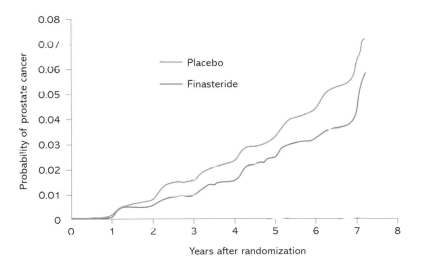

Figure 9.2 Cumulative incidence of prostate cancer confirmed by biopsy for healthy men treated with finasteride or placebo. Source: Thompson et al. 2003.

of this tumor marker for prostate cancer. It seems probable that new tests, or variations of existing ones, will continue to improve the ability of clinicians to distinguish early prostate cancer from benign prostatic conditions, as well as improve outcomes. A possible future approach to screening is shown in Figure 9.3.

Better staging

One of the problems with current management strategies is the inaccuracy of current staging methods. Improved imaging with, for example, TRUS microbubble technology and MRI with gadolinium enhancement or iron filings may improve matters. Moreover, molecular staging, employing polymerase chain reaction technology to identify cells capable of producing messenger RNA coding for PSA, may offer the prospect of detecting microscopic prostate tumor cells in the

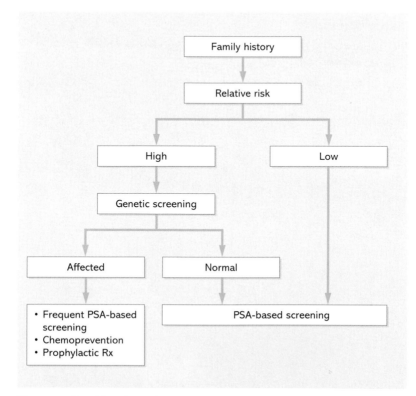

Figure 9.3 Possible scheme for prostate cancer screening in the future.

circulation and thereby avoid futile attempts to eradicate local tumor cells when distant spread has already occurred.

Prognostic indicators

Although earlier detection of prostate cancer will undoubtedly improve the curability of the disease, it also raises the questions of whether a given lesion in an individual patient will or will not progress. Molecular prognostic indicators, such as E-cadherin, anti-cathepsin B and the polycomb group protein EZH2, are currently the subject of intense research, and it seems likely that it will soon be possible to predict more accurately the future behavior of individual prostate cancers. This should facilitate decisions about competing treatment options.

New therapies

For localized prostate cancer, the dominant role of radical prostatectomy and external-beam radiotherapy seems likely to be challenged eventually by newer technologies aimed at ablating the tumor in situ, while minimizing the risks of incontinence and ED. Cryosurgery, high-intensity focused ultrasound and brachytherapy have already been mentioned in this context, and other modalities seem certain to be developed with even less morbidity and perhaps even greater effectiveness. Radical prostatectomy itself may be enhanced by laparoscopic techniques and robotic assistance.

Hormonal manipulation with LHRH analogs seems likely to remain the mainstay of therapy for locally advanced or metastatic disease, though LHRH antagonists and new antiandrogens are currently being evaluated. As antiandrogens are refined, they seem likely to be employed increasingly in earlier stages of the disease, when tumor cell sensitivity to androgen withdrawal may be most pronounced.

Currently, the main problems with hormonal therapy for prostate cancer are the 10–20% of patients who demonstrate hormonal resistance from the time of initiation of therapy, and the remainder, who eventually develop androgen independence after an average 36-month initial response period. Better understanding of the mechanisms by which cells acquire resistance to endocrine treatment is likely to facilitate methods of either delaying or preventing what is currently often an event of ominous prognosis.

Other novel strategies (Table 9.1), such as the development of specific inhibitors for growth factors including, for example, EGF/PDGF, tyrosine kinase and angiogenesis inhibitors, also hold the promise of significant therapeutic advances, perhaps with a lower incidence of side effects.

Agents such as exisulind (Aptosyn), which has pro-apoptotic activity, and trastuzumab (Herceptin), a monoclonal antibody that binds to the *HER-2/neu* receptor, are already being tested in patients with prostate cancer.

The endothelin-A receptor blocker atrasentan has recently been reported to delay time to progression in hormone-refractory prostate cancer.

Prospects for gene therapy. The recent spectacular advances in molecular biology have made the prospect of gene therapy an imminent reality. Gene therapy for prostate cancer is likely to proceed down several avenues, including:

- reasserting control over disturbed cell division mechanisms
- introducing cytotoxic agents specifically into prostate cancer cells leaving normal cells unaffected
- development of vaccines to enhance immunological responses to disseminated prostate cancer cells.

Prostate cancer develops as a result of stepwise activation of oncogenes

TABLE 9.1

Potential therapeutic targets for novel therapies in prostate cancer

• Vitamin D receptor	• Tumor growth factor β
• Bcl-2 (anti-apoptosis gene)	• Microtubule inhibition
• p53	• Angiogenesis inhibition
• Proteosome inhibition	• *HER-2/neu* monoclonal
• Endothelin-A receptor	antibody receptor

and deletion of tumor suppression genes. Potentially, oncogenes could be neutralized or deleted, or tumor suppressor genes reinserted by any of the vector methods currently in development. The unique expression of the PSA promoter area in cells of prostatic origin may provide the vehicle for precise targeting of chemotherapy specifically against prostate cancer cells.

Anti-prostate-cancer vaccines are also now a not-too-distant prospect. Introduction of cytokine genes, such as interleukin-2 or GM-CSF, into harvested prostate cancer cells and subsequent reintroduction into the host has been shown to enhance local and systemic immunological antitumor responses. Dendritic-cell-based therapy may also be proven to be safe and effective.

Concluding thoughts

The prospects for significant advances in the struggle against prostate cancer in the near future are good. To earlier diagnosis, better staging, and more effective and less toxic therapy may be added the possibility of effective chemoprevention. Perhaps in the future it may even be possible to pre-identify the 10% of individuals who are congenitally at risk of eventually developing clinical prostate cancer and thereby target chemoprevention and close surveillance strategies specifically to them. Whatever the future holds, the battle to reduce the morbidity and mortality of prostate cancer seems set to intensify well into the new millennium; family physicians now need to close ranks with urologists and oncologists and strive to ensure that eventual victory is achieved.

Key references

Algaba F, Epstein JI, Aldape HC et al. Assessment of prostate carcinoma in core needle biopsy – definition of minimal criteria for the diagnosis of cancer in biopsy material. *Cancer* 1996;78:376–81.

Carducci MA, Padley RJ, Breul J et al. Effect of endothelin-A receptor blockade with atrasentan on tumor progression in men with hormone-refractory prostate cancer: a randomized, phase II, placebo-controlled trial. *J Clin Oncol* 2003;21:679–89.

Cirantos F, Watson RB, Pinto JE. Finasteride effect on prostatic hyperplasia and prostate cancer. *J Urol Pathol* 1997;6:1–13.

Clark LC, Combs GF Jr, Turnbull BW et al. Effects of selenium supplementation for cancer prevention in patients with carcinoma of the skin. A randomized controlled trial. Nutritional Prevention of Cancer Study Group. *JAMA* 1996:376; 1957–63.

Heinonen OP, Albanes D, Virtamo J et al. Prostate cancer and supplementation with alpha-tocopherol and beta-carotene: incidence and mortality in a controlled trial. *J Natl Cancer Inst* 1998:90:440–6.

Katz AE, Olsson MD, Raffo AJ et al. Molecular staging of prostate cancer with the use of an enhanced reverse transcriptase–PCR assay. *Urology* 1994;43:765–75.

Morris MJ, Scher HI. Novel therapies for the treatment of prostate cancer: current clinical trials and development strategies. *Surg Oncol* 2002;11:13–23.

Nelson PS, Brawer MK. Chemoprevention of prostatic carcinoma. *Urology Int* 1997;4:7–9.

Nelson PS, Gleason TP, Brawer MK. Chemoprevention for prostatic intraepithelial neoplasia. *Eur Urol* 1996;30:269–78.

Ruchlin HS, Pellissier JM et al. An economic overview of prostate carcinoma. *Cancer* 2001;92: 2796–810.

Ryan CW, Stadler WM, Vogelzang NJ. Docetaxel and exisulind in hormone-refractory prostate cancer. *Semin Oncol* 2001;28(4 suppl 15):56–61.

Sanda MG, Ayyagari SR, Jattee EM et al. Demonstration of a rational strategy for human prostate cancer gene therapy. *J Urology* 1994;151: 622–8.

Small EJ, Bok R, Reese DM et al. Docetaxel, estramustine, plus trastuzumab in patients with metastatic androgen-independent prostate cancer. *Semin Oncol* 2001;28(4 suppl 15):71–6.

Thompson I, Goodman PJ, Tangen CM et al. The influence of finasteride on the development of prostate cancer. *N Engl J Med* 2003; 349:215–24.

Valone FH, Small E, MacKenzie M et al. Dendritic cell-based treatment of cancer: closing in on a cellular therapy. *Cancer J* 2001; 7 suppl 2:S53–61.

Varambally S, Dhanasekaran SM, Zhou M et al. The polycomb group protein EZH2 is involved in progression of prostate cancer. *Nature* 2002;419:624–9.

Useful addresses

Prostate Research Campaign UK
Canada House, 272 Field End Road
Eastcote, Middlesex HA4 9NA UK
Tel: 020 8582 0246
info@prostate-research.org.uk
www.prostate-research.org.uk

CancerBACUP
3 Bath Place
Rivington Street
London EC2A 3JR UK
Information service: 020 7613 2121
Free helpline: 0808 800 1234
www.bacup.org.uk

Cancerlink
11–21 Northdown Street
London N1 9BN UK
Free helpline: 0808 808 0000

The Prostate Cancer Charity
3 Angel Walk
London W6 9HX UK
Tel: 020 8222 7622
Fax: 020 8222 7639
Helpline: 0845 300 8383
info@prostate-cancer.org.uk
www.prostate-cancer.org.uk

The Impotence Association
PO Box 10296
London SW1 / 9WH UK
Helpline: 020 8767 7791
www.impotence.org.uk

The Continence Foundation
307 Hatton Square
16 Baldwins Gardens
London EC1N 7RJ UK
Helpline: 020 7831 9831 (9.30 am –
4.30 pm, Monday to Friday)
www.continence-foundation.org.uk

The Men's Health Forum
Tavistock House
Tavistock Square
London WC1H 9HR UK
www.menshealthforum.org.uk

National Prostate Cancer Coalition USA
1154 15th St., NW
Washington, DC 20005 USA
Tel: 202 463 9455
Toll-free: 888 245 9455
Fax: 202 463 9455
info@pcacoalition.org
www.4npcc.org

American Urological Association (AUA)
1120 North Charles Street
Baltimore, MD 21201-5559 USA
Tel: 410 727 1100
www.auanet.org

American Cancer Society (ACS)
1599 Clifton Road
Atlanta, GA 30329 USA
Tel: 800 ACS 2345
www.cancer.org

National Cancer Institute (NCI)
Urologic Oncology Branch
9000 Rockville Pike, Bldg 10, Rm 2B47
Bethesda, MD 20892 USA
Tel: 301 496 6353
www.cancer.gov/cancer_information/
cancer_type/prostate/

Prostate Cancer Education Council
(PCEC)
5299 DTC Blvd, STE 345
Greenwood Village, CO 80111 USA
Tel: 303 316 4685
www.pcaw.com

NW Prostate Institute
1560 N 115th St, STE 209
Seattle, WA 98133 USA
Tel: 206 368 6591
www.prostatecancer.org

Uronet
http://www.phoenix5.org/glossary/
glossary.html

Cancer Research UK
ww.cancerhelp.org.uk

Hormone-Refractory Prostate Cancer
www.hormonerefractorypca.org

Patient UK
www.patient.org.uk

Embarrassing Problems
www.embarrassingproblems.com

Memorial Sloan Kettering Cancer Center
www.mskcc.org/mskcc/html/403.cfm

Brady Urological Institute, Johns
Hopkins University
urology.jhu.edu

Mayo Clinic prostate cancer pages
www.mayoclinic.com/takecharge/
healthdecisionguides/prostatecancer

William Catalona (surgeon who answers
patients' questions on line)
www.drcatalona.com

Index

What the reviewers say:

will likely be read cover to cover in just one or
two sittings by all who are fortunate enough
to obtain a copy

On *Fast Facts – Benign Prostatic Hyperplasia*, 4th edn, in *Doody's Health Sciences Review*, Dec 2002

explains the important facts and demonstrates
the levels of "good practice" that can be achieved

On *Fast Facts – Minor Surgery*,
in *Journal of the Royal Society for the Promotion of Health* 122(3), 2002

a splendid publication

On *Fast Facts – Sexually Transmitted Infections*, in *Journal of Antimicrobial Chemotherapy* 49, 2002

I would highly recommend it
without reservation … 5 stars!

On *Fast Facts – Psychiatry Highlights 2001–02*,
in *Doody's Health Sciences Review*, Sept 2002

I enthusiastically recommend this
stimulating, short book which should
be required reading for all clinicians

On *Fast Facts – Irritable Bowel Syndrome*, in *Gastroenterology* 120(6), 2001

***** outstanding

On *Fast Facts – HIV in Obstetrics and Gynecology*, in *Journal of Pelvic Surgery*, 2001

a gem for family physicians because of its ease
of use and the sophisticated, concise treatment

On *Fast Facts – Epilepsy*, in *American Family Physician* 64(5), 2001

FAST FACTS

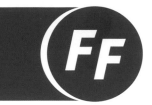

An outstandingly successful independent medical handbook series

Over one million copies sold

- Written by world experts
- Concise and practical
- Up-to-date
- Well structured for ease of reading and reference
- Copiously illustrated with useful photographs, diagrams and charts

Our aim for *Fast Facts* remains the same as ever: to be the world's most respected medical handbook series. Feedback on how to make individual titles even more useful is always welcome (feedback@fastfacts.com).

Some of the *Fast Facts* titles available

Allergic Rhinitis
Benign Gynecological Disease (second edition)
Benign Prostatic Hyperplasia (fourth edition)
Bladder Cancer
Breast Cancer (second edition)
Celiac Disease
Colorectal Cancer (second edition)
Contraception
Dementia
Depression
Diseases of the Testis
Disorders of the Hair and Scalp
Dyspepsia (second edition)
Endometriosis (second edition)
Epilepsy (second edition)
Erectile Dysfunction (third edition)
Gynecological Oncology
Headaches (second edition)
HIV in Obstetrics and Gynecology

Hyperlipidemia (second edition)
Hypertension (second edition)
Inflammatory Bowel Disease
Irritable Bowel Syndrome (second edition)
Menopause
Minor Surgery
Multiple Sclerosis
Osteoporosis (third edition)
Prostate Specific Antigen (second edition)
Psoriasis
Respiratory Tract Infection (second edition)
Rheumatoid Arthritis
Schizophrenia (second edition)
Sexually Transmitted Infections
Soft Tissue Rheumatology
Superficial Fungal Infections
Travel Medicine
Urinary Continence (second edition)
Urinary Stones

Orders

To order via the website, or to find regional distributors, please go to
www.fastfacts.com

For telephone orders, please call 01752 202301 (UK) or
800 538 1287 (North America, toll free)